MW01264359

Self-Defense Why even Bother?

How, why and what to learn to protect yourself

DJ Stephens

R.C.A.T Publishing

Cataloging-in-Publication Data is on file with the Library of Congress

Paperback ISBN 979-8-9866888-0-0

Ebook ISBN 979-8-9866888-1-7

Printed in the USA

Dedication

This book is dedicated to my dad. Not only was he my first self-protection instructor, but without his guidance and supervision, I'm sure that instead of teaching people how to protect themselves against criminals, I would have become a criminal myself.

To my mother for having the wisdom and hindsight to prepare me to deal with all sorts, classes, and races of people. It's because of her that I'm able to do what I do.

Also, to my students. They are the reason that I'm able to wake up in the mornings with a smile on my face. They keep me going. Without them, there would be no me.

Thank you all. You have all my love and gratitude forever!

Contents

Chapter One

Why do "I" even bother?

You're smaller, weaker, and slower than the average bad guy. Why even bother trying to defend yourself? Why not just give up and let the bad guy decide if you or your family live or die? Picture that.

Before we get to the issue at hand, I want to tell you how I became the person I am today. I was born and raised in Washington, D.C. Anyone who knows anything about our nation's capital or any inner-city neighborhood — especially during the '80s or early '90s — knows that things could get pretty rough. There was always a fight. It was nearly impossible to grow up without witnessing or being involved in some level of violence at some point in time during your upbringing.

I was not poor by any stretch of the imagination. I also wasn't rich. I wasn't known as a street-fighting legend. I was affiliated with the neighborhood gangs, but I wasn't in any of the gangs. In D.C., whatever neighborhood you lived in, that was the gang you would be affiliated with. I was just a guy in the neighborhood who knew how to defend himself when needed.

Growing up in the D.C. area at a young age, I realized the importance of knowing how to defend myself. I was always intrigued by martial arts. On the weekends, we watched a television series called "The Action Theater." Every week, this show premiered a different martial arts movie: *Five Deadly Venoms, Enter the Dragon, Fighter in the Wind, The Samurai Warrior,* and so on. Eventually, I was able to convince my mother to enroll me in Jhoon Rhee's Tae kwon do Institute. Jhoon Ree is considered the Godfather of the way American martial arts schools are run today.

My father was a former professional boxer who also trained fighters in the D.C. area at a gym called Finley's Boxing Gym. So, as I was learning to kick from Jhoon Rhee, I was also learning to punch from my dad. It didn't take me long to realize that training for sudden violent situations is unlike training for a boxing match or a Taekwondo tournament.

My brother and I used to do what we called a "play fight." I remember several mornings or nights when my brother would hide behind doors or tables and ambush me when I wasn't expecting it. We would wrestle and fight for minutes at a time. Afterward, we would analyze the different things that happened during the encounter: things we should or shouldn't have done. The next day, I would sneak up on him and repeat the process. We learned to do this without actually hurting each other. We would react to a punch that was thrown as if it were a real punch. We became, I guess you would say, great actors. Little did I know, that training would help me in training years later. We would sometimes pull out boxing gloves and spar, seeing if our strategies worked in somewhat real-time. We would go out and body punch and slap box other guys in the neighborhood. Now and then, an actual fight would break out. Learning to control your emotions was part of the training.

I've always had a passion for teaching. Everything I learned from Jhoon Rhee, my dad, and the training with my brother, I would go out and teach and instruct anyone interested in learning. Teaching made me better at doing. To this day, I can't own a technique or a skill unless I've taught it. Pretty soon, I found myself training younger kids in the neighborhood. I turned my grandmother's garage into a

fighting gym with a punching bag, speed bag, weights, and all. Watching the young ones get better quickly became the highlight of my evenings. To this day, nothing else gives me more fulfillment than watching my students grow. I often tell people that I am passionate about martial arts and that teaching is my purpose.

In my mid-teens, my mother wanted me to have the same advantages, training, and schooling as the kids who were brought up in more upper-class neighborhoods, so she enrolled me in a private school. There, I was exposed to and made friends with a variety of different kids from all sorts of backgrounds and cultures: upper class, middle class, lower class, white, Hispanic, Asian, etc. Although I went back and graduated from a D.C. public high school, Theodore Roosevelt, I remained friends and stayed in contact with a few of my private school buddies even to this day. Soon after graduation, I moved to Bethesda, Maryland, to an area called Glen Echo. Glen Echo is pretty much as upscale as you can get in the Maryland area. My family had held on to the property that was awarded to us after slavery. That was where I lived for the next fifteen years. The reason why I bring all that up is that no matter what school I attended, what friends I made, or which environment I lived in, the need to know how to protect

myself was still important, if for no other reason but peace of mind.

Over the years, I've trained in many martial arts systems: Taekwondo, Krav Maga, Jiu Jitsu, Boxing, etc. The training I received in those systems helped me to prepare for violent encounters, and now I want to pass my knowledge on to you. However, the art or system is not nearly as important as the training or mindset. What I would like to teach you is what I have learned, observed, and trained in for over thirty years. This is not a book to teach you to punch here and kick there. This is not a book to go over pressure points or vulnerable areas in the human body. Although those things are important, this book will help you understand self-protection, not only how, but also what, from whom to train, but maybe even more importantly, why should you even bother?

Chapter Two

What Does It Even Mean? Why Even Bother?

What is self-defense? Self-defense is defined as a counter-measure that involves defending the health and well-being of oneself or another from harm. Legally, it is described as the right to prevent suffering from violence through the use of a sufficient level of counteracting force or violence. In the streets, self-defense is simply called "doing what you gotta do." It's important to know that what you may consider self-defense may not hold up in a court of law or a jury of your peers. On the one hand, it is imperative that you know the law before you act. Then there is also the popular phrase that says, "It's better to be judged by twelve than to be carried by six."

Note: For the remainder of this book, I will not use the term "self-defense." Instead, I will use the term "self-protection."

I have a company called CDK. CDK is an acronym for Confidence During Kaos. Yes, I spell Chaos with a K :). That name was given to me by a friend who came up with it. That is my mission exactly: to instill confidence in my students, the confidence to walk down the street and go about their lives knowing that they can protect themselves. Ninety percent of the students that call or come into my classes all have similar stories: *I work at night, sometimes I'm alone, and I don't feel safe. There's been a rise in crime in my neighborhood, and I need to know how to protect myself. I work in security or law enforcement, and learning self-protection is important. Learning self-protection is something that I've always wanted to do. Now that I have more time, I feel that it is better late than never.* In other words, they are looking for confidence in a chaotic world. The creator of Krav Maga, Imi Lichtenfeld, said, "You must learn to defend yourself so that one may walk in peace."

It is hard for me to imagine what it must feel like to walk around in public without having any idea of what to do if a violent situation were to happen. Violence can happen anywhere: on the Metro, in a restaurant, and nowadays, even in the workplace. Whitney Young, an American Civil Rights leader, once said, "It is better to be prepared for an opportunity and not have one than to have an opportunity and not be prepared." I paraphrase that quote by saying, "It is better to be prepared for a situation and never have one than to have a situation and not be prepared." Being prepared is what self-protection training is all about.

Being prepared

As I said before, self-protection training is different from sports training. Sports training gets you ready for an event that you know will happen, expect to happen, and even want to happen. Self-protection training prepares you for an event that is just the opposite. You do not know if it will happen. You do not know when it will happen. You hope and pray that it never does. I often tell my students, that for an hour or two that they will be on the training floor, to try to mentally put themselves in an entirely different frame of mind. Often, this frame of mind is quite different from their natural personality. In Krav Maga, the goal is to become aggressive. At CDK, we add what we call "controlled aggression." Pure aggression is what I would equate to an out-of-control forest fire. Controlled aggression is a flamethrower in the hands of someone who knows how to operate it. Learning how to use a flamethrower is something that has to be taught. The art of self-protection has to be taught as well.

Although we call it unarmed self-protection, no human being is born unarmed. Every human is armed with abilities, attributes, and body parts to protect themselves from incoming attacks. Just with the hand alone, you have your knuckles, your back fist, your fingertips, the ridge of your hand, the blade side of your hand, the palm heel of your hand, your thumb knuckle, and a few more. That's just your hand. You have weapons all over your body, not to mention your best weapon of all: the six inches in between your ears. Just like with a flamethrower, the more comfortable you are using your weapons, the more confident you will be in a situation.

The art of self-protection is the God-given right of all living creatures. All of us have been given the tools. We all have the ability. Self-protection training will give us the skill. This skill comes from hours and hours of beating on your craft. In this case, the craft or art of self-protection.

Oh, that wouldn't work.

That would get you killed.

No one reacts like that.

I've heard every excuse in the book from naysayers and critics of self-protection techniques and strategies. But when it comes to self-protection, there's one thing these naysayers fail to understand: the element of surprise.

When you train for self-protection, you have to take into consideration that your attacker or adversary does not know what you are about to attempt. I can tell you countless stories of students, friends, and acquaintances that were put into the unfortunate position of having to defend themselves and were able to do so. I just watched a story about a dramatic moment of an eleven-year-old who was able to fight off a kidnapper with a knife in Florida. The kidnapper pulled up to a bus stop where the girl was waiting for a bus early in the morning. He jumped out of the car with a knife and ran over to grab her. Fortunately, she was paying attention and saw him coming and started to run away. He caught up with her, and she landed a kick, screamed, and got away. The kidnapper counted on the little girl freezing and easily taking her away. One of our affiliate schools has a member that recently had to fight off a carjacker/kidnapper with a gun. The student had just pulled up and was getting his daughter out of the car. A dude approached him and demanded that he give up his car keys. Any other time, he would have complied, but his daughter was in the car. When he told the bad guy that his daughter was in the car, he was still persistent. He wanted both the car and the child. Our affiliate member was forced to fight the assailant for the gun. Fortunately, he was on the phone with his partner at the time, who quickly called the police. He was able to control the gunman's wrist and keep himself and his daughter out of the line of fire until the gunman heard the sirens and fled the scene. Then there's the cab driver who was taken to a fake address. Two bad guys had planned to not only rob him but also kill him and dump his body at the scene. They did not know that the cab driver was carrying a firearm of his own. He was able to defend himself by killing one of the bad guys and wounding the other. Later, the police found out that both of the bad guys had been involved in several homicides and had warrants for their arrest.

In none of these cases did the bad guys think that their prey would fight back. They did not think that because, normally, people don't. Most will do nothing. Some will freeze. Then some will deny what is happening until it's too late. It's said that you will always do what you are trained to do. If you are trained to do nothing, then you will do nothing.

Dreams don't work unless you do something, and neither will your training if you don't have any.

Chapter Three

Three Types of Violent Encounters

I would like to take this time to show respect to all of the self-protection gurus that I have followed over the years. Authors and teachers like Roy Miller, Tim Larkin, and Tony Brewer have all created countless books, podcasts, blogs, articles, etc. I could only hope to one day be considered or even mentioned in the same sentence as some of these gentlemen. That being said, the things that I'm speaking of do not come from any book. They're not from data or research or any police or prison files. They come from real-life experiences. These are things that I have witnessed or been a part of. The things that I'm explaining to you are not debatable. With that being said, there are three types of violent encounters that I have witnessed or been a part of.

The first self-protection scenario is the planned fight. From a legal standpoint, this is probably the hardest scenario to prove that you acted legally in a court of law. Although it may be the most difficult to prove legally, it is most definitely one that I would prefer if I was forced to pick one to be in. What is a fight? A fight—a physical fight—is what I describe or define as when two people or a group of people decide to settle their differences physically or violently. Planned fights happen every day. They were surely popular back in grade school. Just think about the three o'clock schoolyard brawl. Everyone knew who was going to fight and where they were going to fight. They even knew who was expected to win which is why I said it would be the one that I would prefer. The planned fight is the encounter that most young men train for. It is primitive but, believe it or not, sometimes necessary. We will discuss social and asocial violence, but for now, just know that for some, the planned fight today may help you avoid the second and third types of violent encounters later.

The second type of violent encounter is the unplanned flight. You did not know that it was going to happen. You did not plan for it to happen. You may not have even wanted it to happen but you found yourself in a situation that you deemed unavoidable. A good example of this would be the famous bar fight analogy. A lot of self-protection lessons and classes start with, "So you're at the bar and..." An unplanned fight is a fight when you may have felt you needed to defend your honor, the honor of someone you care about, or maybe you just had to defend yourself or a loved one from bodily harm. This type of self-protection situation may be easier to explain in a court of law than the first, but it can still and very likely get you into bad legal trouble. This type of encounter is not the type of encounter that women usually train for. This sort of violent encounter is what men, both young and even seasoned, train for. This is an encounter that you can usually see coming. There is some sort of buildup, usually an argument, a discussion that turned into an argument, an accidental bump against the shoulder, a stomp on the foot without an "excuse me" to follow, or just a stare-down that went on for too long. When most men think about self-protection training, this is the one that they visualize.

The third type of violent encounter is not only the worst, it is the one that you don't want to be in. This is a sudden, violent attack, an ambush. You did not plan to fight. There was no buildup. There was no warning. The chances are you weren't ready and were caught totally off guard. Legally, if you are the victim of a sudden violent attack and you defend yourself, as long as you know how to articulate what happened, you will probably be able to walk away with no jail time. I hear a lot of self-protection teachers and instructors talk about things that you can do in a self-protection situation. *Plant your feet to get power in your punch.* This is not for a violent sudden attack. *Pinpoint your strikes. Go for the eyes, the throat, and the groin.* Not in the sudden violent attack. *Use proper technique.* This does not apply to the sudden violent attack. In a sudden violent attack, you are off balance and you can't plant your feet. You are surprised, so you can't pinpoint your strikes. You can't use the proper technique because, by the time you are even able to think, the encounter is usually over. This is the encounter that most women train for. Women worry about the walk to the car or the run in the woods (don't run in the woods). The truth of the matter is that this is the type that everyone should train for. The problem is that people don't know how to train for it. Some think they don't need to. Others think they are already trained for it, but they're not. Then some don't even think they can. Most say, "Why even bother?"

Chapter Four

Reasons NOT to defend yourself

Although this book is primarily written to give you reasons to defend yourself and how to train for it, it's important for me to first give you a few reasons to *not* defend yourself. I have given a few quotes by some other self-protection gurus that I mentioned in the previous chapter. *"Violence is rarely the answer, but when it is, it's the only answer."* —Tim Larkin, When Violence is the Answer.

Violence is sometimes the answer, but what about when it isn't? If I know how to defend myself, why shouldn't I do it?

Any time a prospective student calls and wants to take classes, I always ask them why they want to learn Krav Maga. This particular lady called me and said that she wanted to learn how to defend herself because she gets verbally harassed a lot and she wants to be able to say something back to them. If the situation escalates, she wants to know what to do to defend herself.

While I have sympathy for women and other people who regularly experience street harassment, that is a terrible reason to want to learn Krav Maga. <u>It's always better to just walk, or even run away when you can</u>. I know there are a lot of women out there who want to be able to do anything they want to do, go anywhere they want to go, and say anything they want to say, but in the real world, these are all terrible decisions. I know there are a lot of dudes out there who have egos and pride. There are also a lot of dudes that sleep with tombstones over their heads because they could've and should've walked away but didn't. There are also a lot of people in prison for the same reason. Here are three good reasons not to defend yourself or attempt to defend yourself.

The first reason you should always try to avoid having to defend yourself is that there is no guarantee that you're going to win. My father always said that there is nobody in this world that can beat everybody. There's always somebody better than you. The person that you happen to get into a confrontation with might be that person. As they say in the streets, "You don't want that smoke." Sometimes, losing a fight means getting a broken nose. Sometimes, it's a black eye. Sometimes, it's just your ego that is damaged. However, sometimes, it can mean your life. You just never know how a violent confrontation is going to end. We would like to think that it would end with the bad guy laying on the ground saying he's sorry and you just walking away with your chest out with no one being seriously hurt. However, in reality, that may not be the case. The bad guy may not even have the intention of taking your life or causing you serious bodily harm. His intentions may have just been to give you a minor injury but you fall, hit your head on the curb, and...

The second reason to try to avoid a situation or violent encounter is because of what I always teach my students. You should always assume your attacker has a weapon and a friend. I have been training in martial arts and self-protection for most of my life. A lot of people would say, "If somebody has a knife, then I should be able to defend myself." If someone had a knife, even with all my training, there is a high chance that I would be seriously harmed or even killed. A lot of people would say, "If it's multiple attackers, I should be OK." If there are multiple attackers, there's a big chance that I will be seriously harmed or even killed. Although, I could probably defend myself better than a person who has had no training, if my attacker has a knife or I am attacked by a group of people, the odds are still in their favor.

The third reason to always avoid a confrontation is the legal and psychological ramifications of winning the fight. I know you may be thinking that winning the fight will make you feel good, but there is more to it than just that particularly if you are a good person. Good people generally don't like to hurt people, and as I mentioned earlier, you never know how the fight may end. You may end up permanently injuring or even killing the other person, only to later find out that it was just a big misunderstanding. You have hired a lawyer, and you're possibly facing jail time. At the end of the day, it is just not worth it.

Once again, I'm only referring to the situations that can be avoided.

"It's better to avoid than to run. It is better to run than to de-escalate. It is better to de-escalate than to fight. It's better to fight than to die." —Roy Miller, Facing violence.

Chapter Five

I Don't Want to Fight You

I'd like to share with you a question that someone had on one of my YouTube videos. He said, "Here's my struggle: I've been doing Krav Maga for six months before the pandemic. I've recently taken up private sessions with my instructor, and I've discovered something. I am a very devout spiritual Christian, and because of this, I find it very hard to be aggressive when I spar. Behind the fear of me getting hit, there's the fear of me hitting others or potentially hurting them. I discovered this for the first time when I sparred with a fellow student. In short, he was being an asshole, and he was throwing palm heel strikes at my unprotected nose, so out of fear, I did an improvised eye gouge and nearly blinded him. I mean, it stopped the fight, but at the same time, I didn't mean to hurt him. My question is this: For my faith and the love of fellow human beings, how can I develop the mindset of being aggressive and violent as a means to protect myself and others while at the same time not hurting my attacker or sinking to their level?"

"I don't even call it violence when it comes to self-protection, I call it intelligence." — Malcolm X.

The subject of violence as it pertains to self-protection has been discussed and debated for years. When should you use violence? Should you use violence? How should you use violence? Is it okay to use violence? The truth of the matter is that a lot of people find it very difficult to intentionally harm another person, even when they have been put in situations where that is the most intelligent thing to do. It has a lot to do with a person's upbringing, belief system, and even state of mind. In this segment, I'm going to break down three reasons you should defend yourself.

The first reason why you should use self-protection is when, as brother Malcolm would say, it's intelligent to do so. Let's say somebody is punching you or about to punch you in the face. The only way you feel that you're going to stop him is to kick him in the groin. That would be intelligent. Let's say a criminal is about to sexually assault you, and the only way you feel you can stop that assault from happening is to pull out your gun and shoot. That would be intelligent. You are a police officer, and someone pulls a gun on you and fires, so you fire back. That would be intelligent.

The first reason you should defend yourself is that it is the most intelligent thing in that particular circumstance. How can you choose not to stop someone from hurting you? How can you choose not to stop someone from killing you? How do you choose not to stop someone from harming your loved one? Don't be mistaken. I would rather rectify the situation without having to defend myself violently, but when it comes to self-protection, it's not about violence. It's about intelligence.

The second thing you should think about as to why you should be okay with using self-protection or violence is that your intentions are good. Let's go back to that example of somebody punching you in the face. The only thing you can do to stop them is to kick them in the stones. You intend to stop the attack. You may not dislike the person. You may not have any ill will toward the person. Your intentions are good because it is good to stop someone from punching you in the face. You shouldn't get your intentions confused with your emotions. Now, we can get into talking about the lizard brain and survival or monkey brain and emotion, but just know that when your intentions are good (you're trying to defend yourself or your loved one), then your emotions are not what's important. It's easy to get your emotions and feelings confused with your intent. If you don't like someone, that does not give you the right to harm them in any way. In my opinion, it is only okay and even justified when they are in the process of harming you or a loved one and your intention is to stop them.

The third reason why you should defend yourself is that you're given no other choice. This is a situation when you have exhausted all of your options. You could not avoid the situation. You could not run from the situation. You could not de-escalate the situation. The only options are to defend yourself and deal with the situation or let them decide what happens to you. The only way you can deal with this situation is to intelligently defend yourself. Sometimes, you can go through all your options in a matter of seconds, like in the third type of violent encounter – the sudden violent encounter. Sometimes it's a buildup and you go through your options slowly. On either account, you have exhausted your possibilities and you feel that you have to use the reasonable amount of force that you deem necessary to defend yourself.

Why Not Just Buy a Gun?

One of the most popular debates around the topic of un-armed self-protection is armed self-protection. Why not just buy a gun?

Let me preface this by saying that this is a touchy subject, especially with all the recent and senseless mass shootings happening all around our country. The question of gun ownership is a debate that has been going on for years and will no doubt continue for many more. Politicians, from local city council members to the president of the United States, are voted in or out depending on which side of the feud they support. I am not here to debate whether or not you should be pro-gun or anti-gun. I am here to give you my opinion and expertise on the best ways for mentally stable and law-abiding citizens to defend themselves if the situation presents itself. Let's start with a simple question: should you own and carry a firearm for self-protection?

Whether or not you decide to carry a firearm depends on different variables, including the laws in your jurisdiction, your ability to use a firearm, and most importantly, your mental state at the time. But should you own a gun for self-protection? My answer is yes. Here are three reasons to support my answer:

First, the bad guys have guns. I have trained extensively in several different martial arts and self-protection systems.

Don't be delusional into thinking that any of these systems will fend off a bad guy who has a gun and is willing to use it. As I've stated before, I have been studying and training in Krav Maga for fourteen years and counting at the time of writing this book. I am a 2nd degree black belt in Krav Maga, a black belt in Taekwondo, and I'm presently learning Jiu Jitsu. Krav Maga is known for its proficiency in gun disarming and takeaways. I have done gun disarms under staged stress, fatigue, and injury. I'm pretty sure that I have practiced gun takeaways well over a thousand times from different angles and situations. With all that training, if someone were to pull a gun on me and I went for the takeaway, I would give myself no more than a 50-50 chance of survival.

Now, of course, a 50 percent chance is much better than a zero percent survival rate, but even with all my training, it can go either way. I don't think any martial arts or self-protection expert would disagree with me when I say that no matter how skilled or badass you may be, if your adversary has a firearm and you don't, then you are at a grave disadvantage. One of my favorite rap lyrics from the late great Biggie Smalls was, *"Picture me being scared when a N#gg* that breathes the same air as me. Picture me being shook when we can both pull burners and let the mother f**king beef cook."* When I bring up that line, some people will bring up the fact that Biggie was shot and killed. They are missing the point of what I'm saying, which is that if the bad guy has a gun and so do I, then I, at least, have a fighter's chance of survival. They are also missing two other key points: A) When Biggie was shot, he wasn't armed; and B) Even if he was, it may not have saved him. There were a lot of circumstances around his murder that were complicated and still unsolved. Nevertheless, I still believe in those particular lyrics.

Second, guns are the weapon of choice in the time that we live in. Thousands of years ago, before guns were invented, swords were the weapon of choice. If you did not own a sword or did not know how to use a sword, you were at the bottom of the village. Not only could you not defend yourself, but, more importantly, you could not protect the ones you love. Imagine laying in your hut with your wife and kids and a scavenger walks in with a sword and you didn't have one. Nowadays, having a sword is a useless waste of time. Why? Because even Sir Lancelot himself, with all his shining armor, would be defenseless if he came upon a knight with a gun. (Believe it or not, there's still a debate as to which is better between a gun and a sword. Go figure.)

Not only do I feel that it is important that you have the weapon of choice of the time, but it is also important that you know how to use the weapon of choice at the time. A sword is useless to a knight who cannot wield it. A gun is useless to a good guy who cannot shoot it. Just like with the sword, learning to use a firearm takes practice—less practice than with a sword, but still, practice. How can you practice learning to use a firearm if you don't own a firearm? Yeah, of course, you can go to the shooting range and rent a firearm, but it's nothing like having your own. Not to mention, after a few visits and renting at the gun range financially, it stops making sense.

Third, a gun is a deterrent. Here is the truth of the matter: if you are truly a good person, you don't want to ever have to harm another person. You would rather just walk away. A gun could very well give you that option. I have personally been in and around situations that could have easily escalated to violence but were quickly de-escalated when just the handle of a gun was shown. A gun is a deterrent.

So, why even bother with self-protection when guns exist in the world? Why even bother learning to protect yourself without a firearm? The answers are easy. Maybe you are unable to get to your firearm. Maybe using your firearm is well over the amount of force needed to defend yourself. I'll discuss that scenario more later on. For now, I want to offer an example from one of the most armed subsets of our population: law enforcement officers.

Several law enforcement officers come into my school for training to learn Krav Maga. I also have trained with several highly decorated law enforcement officers in Jiu Jitsu. Whether we're training in Krav Maga, Jiu Jitsu, boxing, or even Taekwondo, all of these officers have one thing in common. They all carry a firearm. So why are they learning and training in unarmed combat? Because sometimes getting to your weapon, even when it's on your side, may not be an immediate option. Even among law enforcement officers, this is true. I have studied countless videos where an officer was ambushed and had to use both hands to defend him or herself and could not reach for their sidearm.

Second, at the time of an altercation, you may not have your firearm. Listen, I don't care how much you love your guns. No one has their gun available to them twenty-four hours a day, seven days a week, and there are places where you cannot lawfully take your firearm. Think about airports, nightclubs and bars, churches, and government buildings. These are places where you cannot lawfully take your firearm, but we all know violence happens there anyway. Most establishments that sell alcohol don't allow you to have a firearm, but the chance of violence happening in a place where alcohol is sold is still high. We all know violence is likely to occur in such places. Do you want to walk around paranoid because you don't have your weapon?

Do you want to be unable to defend yourself and your family because you can't get to your weapon? Or do you want to become a weapon if need be? The point is, as much as we want to believe they are, firearms are not the be-all and end-all. If you truly want to be able to defend yourself in any situation, you must learn to defend yourself without the use of a firearm.

Whether or not you decide to own or carry a firearm is totally up to you (and, of course, the state in which you live). I am not here to judge. I'm just here to inform you and give you the best information to help you decide what course to take to be able to protect yourself and your loved ones. *Confidence comes from discipline and training.* —Robert Kiyosaki. So, whichever decision you make, have the discipline and get the training.

Chapter Six

There must be Another Way

The consensus I get from a lot of people is the pushback on why they should have to do any of these things in the first place. Why should they have to check with the local police department or research crimes in the area? Why should they have to learn to use their voice to get out of the situation? Why should they have to dress a certain way? Well, honestly, you don't have to do any of those things. You can just go about your business and either pretend, ignore, or remain oblivious to what's going on in the world every day. But pretending, ignoring, and remaining oblivious will not help you avoid situations that could happen to you. *"I'm not here to tell you how to handle the world the way you wished it was. I'm here to help you deal with the world the way it really is."* – Tim Larkin

Guns are popular, but they are not and cannot be the only way. In this chapter, I will discuss alternatives to gun use that can help keep you safe.

There are some methods that every self-protection instructor teaches in their workshops, schools, classes, and seminars:

Awareness: keeping both eyes open and being aware of the people around you.

De-escalation: knowing what to say, what not to say, and how to say it.

The buddy system (especially when it comes to young females and college settings).

Knowing your surroundings and knowing where you are.

Repetition is the mother of skill, and these things are worth repeating. That being said, I want to get more in-depth or even go in another direction because sometimes avoiding, de-escalating, the buddy system, or even knowing where you are is not enough if you don't know what any of those things even mean. Let's talk about avoiding a situation and the methods we use.

First, let's talk about how to carry yourself.

Knowing how you carry yourself is crucial when it comes to avoiding a situation. When I say how you carry yourself, I'm talking about the way you walk, the way you dress, and even the way you look at another person. These details matter.

I've seen both men and women walk down the street with absolutely no sign of confidence whatsoever. Shoulders hunched. Heads down. It's almost like they are trying to become invisible, and that's because they are. The funny thing is that these people aren't always people who have low confidence. Sometimes it's just the opposite. It is a common thought that if you seem harmless, then no one would want to harm you. If I don't bother them, they won't bother me. If I don't say anything to them, they won't say anything to me. If I don't look at them, they won't look at me.

I'm here to tell you that this is wrong, wrong, wrong. Predators, i.e., people who are looking to start trouble, are looking for an easy win. Walking without confidence doesn't keep you hidden from predators. It makes you stand out to them as an easy mark. By contrast, walking with your chest up not only says *I am confident*, but it tells the world *I am ready*. Walking with your head up says, *I am not only confident but I am observant.* Being able to look a person in the eye (although there is a timeframe) is saying, *I see you*.

The way you dress matters. Yes, I know you should be able to dress any way you want. For that matter, you should be able to walk any way that you want. I am not going to get into what you should and shouldn't be able to do. I am talking about what you can do to avoid a situation. One of those things is dressing appropriately. For example, if you're wearing shoes that you are unable to run in and someone wants to chase you, you become a target. If you're wearing clothes that you can't move around in, and someone wants to attack you, you become a target. Sometimes the colors that you wear in certain neighborhoods make you a target. More on that shortly. Listen, I'm not saying that you have to walk tough and rough or dress like a badass to avoid a confrontation. What I am saying is, if you want to know some small things you can do now so that you won't have to deal with big situations later, the way you carry yourself and what you wear is one of them.

Second, let's talk about using your voice.

There are several de-escalation tactics, but right now I just want to focus on the importance of using your voice and making noise. Not just any noise—LOUD noise. I have been teaching my students to use their voices for as long as I've been teaching. I tell them that using their voice, especially in a violent or potentially violent situation, has so many different benefits. It gives you power. In traditional martial arts, they call it your chi. It brings attention to the situation. It tells the world that you didn't start this fight, but you want everybody to know that you're in one. It also increases the chances that someone may come to your assistance.

I encourage anyone reading this book to check out a video called, *Secrets to avoid getting mugged: A veteran thief reveals all*, which profiles career criminals. The documentary interviews prisoners who give people advice on what to do and what not to do to defend themselves and their belongings against robbers and stick-up kids. One particular criminal interviewed was what we call a "stick-up kid." The first thing I remember him saying is that he looks for people who are not paying attention. If he notices they aren't paying attention, he can close the distance and get to them before they can react. I thought, *CHECK, I teach that*. The second thing I remember him saying is that most people would be better off just giving him what he wants. Once he decides that he is going to try to take something like a purse, wallet, or car key, he will do so relentlessly and violently if need be. If you gave him what he wanted voluntarily, he would not need violence. Things are just things.

They can be replaced. I thought, *CHECK, I teach that*. (Now, of course, if a perpetrator wants something more than just your purse or wallet—more than just something that can be replaced—that's another story. In this particular context, I am talking about physical objects that can be replaced).

This brings me to the third thing this career criminal said in Muggers Tell All. It was a simple question asked by the interviewer: who do you rob more? Men or women? I always pose this question to my students in my workshops. Oftentimes, the majority of students come up with the same answer: women. But the criminal's answer was, "men." When the interviewee looked surprised, the career criminal explained to him that the reason why he robbed men more was that women scream. I said *CHECK, and double CHECK, I teach that!*

The average woman instinctively has no problem using her voice to scream when she's startled. I try to channel that into speaking with authority. Speak loudly, along with screaming or yelling, if necessary. Predators and would-be attackers tend to not want to draw attention to the situation. Knowing how to use your voice is important when it comes to not only avoiding a situation but also getting out of it.

Next, let's talk about knowing where you are.

An attack can happen anywhere. We are seeing more and more videos of attacks happening in upscale neighborhoods, public places where other people are around, places where you wouldn't think that it would happen, and places where you think that you would be safe. That being said, be aware of where you are. Are you in an area where there are a lot of carjackings? Are you in an area where there are a lot of assaults? Are you in a place where kidnappings occur? Are you in gang territory? Knowing the area and what's going on in the area could help you be more aware. Have you done your research when you move or are thinking about moving to an area? Have you checked with the local police department on crime in the area? In this day and age, information on particular areas is just a "Hey Google" moment away. Have you done some research on what is going on in that area if you are going on vacation or visiting? Is it a high crime area or a low crime area? When I go on vacation, I like to know where I am and even where I'm going. I like Jamaica, for example. When I go to Ocho Rios or to Negril, which tends to be safer, I am in a different mindset (although I am still aware) than when I go to Kingston, which has a higher crime rate. I live in Washington, D.C. When I'm in the D.C. area and I am driving through Bethesda, Maryland, a high-end, ritzy part of town, I have a different mindset (although I stay aware) than I do when I'm driving through Southeast D.C., which is a higher-crime area. Know where you are.

I'll just add this one to the list. Know how to leave. You know how you got to a certain location. Do you know how to get away? My sister offers a great example of what I'm talking about. Back in the day, she used to frequent clubs and would always look for the exit doors when she first arrived. She always wanted to know how to get out if she had to. This can be applied inside a building or to an outside space as well. Knowing how to get away, knowing the surroundings, and knowing where you are could be an alternative to having to defend yourself in the first place. That is a form of protecting yourself. Bruce Lee would call it *"The art of fighting without fighting."*

Chapter Seven

The Arts: Which One is the best?

Finding a self-protection or martial arts school is a lot different today than it was when I was growing up. Back then, if you wanted to learn to defend yourself, you just went to your local boxing gym or took some form of Karate. I think everybody I know has taken Karate, Kung Fu, or Taekwondo at least once in their childhood. We also used to watch Bruce Lee, Jackie Chan, and action theater movies. Every movie had pretty much the same theme: who's fighting style is the best?

We've come a long way since then. The real turning point came in 1993 with the introduction of the UFC (Ultimate Fighting Championship). The UFC changed everything. It introduced a fighting style called Jiu Jitsu and it took the world by storm. Since then, other arts have risen to combat or enhance the teachings of Jiu Jitsu. From there, we have the creation or evolution of what they call reality self-protection. What this means is that things that they teach in a lot of the traditional martial arts systems do not work in real street situations.

The truth is, no matter what you train in, traditional martial arts, Asian martial arts, Brazilian martial arts, or reality self-protection, they all have been watered down from their original state. Finding a legitimate place to train nowadays when you are training for street violence is harder than getting out of a Gracie chokehold. Even Jiu Jitsu is watered down from its original form when there was less emphasis on sports and tournaments. At the end of the day, it matters less about what art you're learning and more about the instructors teaching the art.

Honestly, the more mainstream the system or school is, the more watered-down it has probably become. Why? It's because a lot of people really don't like to train, at least not in the way that will give them the best results. It's like going to a gym or finding a workout. In today's world, the workouts that people tend to lean toward are anything that makes working out look easy. The online cardio workout where everyone is smiling and having so much fun. The weightlifting system doesn't require you to lift weights.

They even have machines now that claim to get you in great shape and burn body fat while you sit down. This is the world that we live in. Martial arts, i.e., self-protection systems, are no different. There are countless training systems available, but the training or art forms that I am going to discuss in this chapter are the art forms that I have either studied personally, have dabbled in, or that I have black belts in. I'll also say that I am going to speak about these arts based on what they are in their purest forms, not the commercialized versions. When it comes to their level of efficiency, I'm speaking of the average practitioner, not necessarily the higher 15th and 20th-degree black belts. After all, if you are a high-level practitioner in any reputable art, you should have no problem defending yourself.

Jiu Jitsu

Jiu Jitsu, or to be more specific, Brazilian Jiu Jitsu, or BJJ, is a martial art and combat sport based on ground fighting and submission holds. It focuses on the skill of taking an opponent to the ground, controlling one's opponent, gaining a dominant position, and using some techniques to force the opponent into submission via joint locks or choke holds.

Jiu Jitsu gained popularity during the first UFC tournaments in the early '90s and was put on the map by a young competitor named Royce Gracie. Royce ran through the tournaments with seemingly no effort against other competitors who were bigger, stronger, and perceived to be better than he was. I have fond, personal memories of watching this. The first UFC was introduced to the world as a no holds barred, no-rules tournament to find out which style was the best. I can remember the exact place, time, and television I was watching at the time. All I could say after watching him fight was "Holy shit! What just happened?" He walked through all of his competitors, who were all bigger and stronger, in a matter of seconds. Today, we know Royce Gracie was one of the few, if not the only practitioner in that tournament, who was a high-level martial artist. However, back then, he single-handedly changed the world of martial arts right before our eyes.

After its UFC introduction, Jiu Jitsu was marketed as the most effective fighting system of all time. Countless numbers of black and white beta and VHS tapes of instructors and other martial artists who challenged the founders of the system were defeated one by one. At that time, there was no internet and YouTube didn't exist. So, the only way to learn Jiu Jitsu was by ordering tapes and having them sent to your house. It was rare to find a Jiu Jitsu school in any area. But as popularity grew, that soon changed and Jiu Jitsu schools began popping up all over the country. The marketing slogan for Jiu Jitsu in the '90s and early 2000s was simple: "90 percent of street fights end up on the ground." Soon, any UFC mixed martial artist who did not have at least some sort of Jiu Jitsu knowledge before they entered the cage-fighting octagon was committing what we called cage suicide. To this day, it is probably the fastest-growing martial arts/self-protection system of all time. I have been taking Jiu Jitsu on and off for some years now. To roll (spar) with a high level or sometimes even a mid-level practitioner can be horrifying. If your ego is not in check, you probably won't make it past the first month. That's one of the reasons why the turnover rate in this martial art is so high. No matter who you are or what stand-up systems you have become proficient in, you have to be willing to (pardon the pun) start from the ground.

But does it work?

Is it effective in a real situation? Jiu Jitsu is unquestionably effective in a real situation. According to Joe Rogan, commentator of UFC and Jiu Jitsu black belt, the average purple belt in Jiu Jitsu is an assassin on the street. This is true because the average person walking down the street, or the average criminal even, is unfamiliar with defending themselves against joint locks and chokes, especially while on the ground. If you are at least a purple belt or a high-level blue belt for that matter (purple belt being the third stage of Jiu Jitsu and blue belt being the second), you will have a high success rate of being able to defend yourself in a confrontation but there is a catch. Just like with anything, there are pros and cons to everything.

The pros

Jiu Jitsu is a highly effective fighting system. It is undoubtedly the most effective fighting system that emphasizes fighting on the ground, and one of the best qualities of Jiu Jitsu is the system's training methods. Unlike other striking arts, you can practice Jiu Jitsu at full speed and force without causing injury to your training partner. Jiu Jitsu focuses on joint locks and chokes. Unlike what you see in movies, breaking a joint takes a certain amount of pressure if it is not blunt force. Your training partner can 'tap,' which is what Jiu Jitsu teaches you to do when you are experiencing pain before injury occurs. Chokes also don't happen as easily as you see in the movies. So, if you find yourself in a choke hold, you can tap before you lose consciousness. This sounds like a brutal way of training, but it is actually quite safe. Jiu Jitsu practitioners suffer fewer injuries than most other fighting arts. I often tell my students when I speak of Jiu Jitsu that if you are a Jiu Jitsu student, you don't 'think' that you can get an arm bar or choke hold on a person successfully, you *know* it. When you are getting trained in Jiu Jitsu, you are often training at full speed, and they don't typically give it to you. Students earn it. So, when you've 'tapped' someone, you know you've done it. That realization alone gives you extreme confidence in your abilities. I will repeat this several times: the way you carry yourself is a huge part of not having to engage in a violent confrontation in the first place. Nothing will help you to carry yourself more positively than confidence.

The cons

"Ninety percent of street fights end up on the ground." Even if you believe that, which I don't, 100 percent of fights start standing up. In my experience, the 90 percent ground rule is actually not true. I would argue that going to the ground is not always the best option. Now, it may work well in a situation when one person decides to settle their differences physically with another person, but what happens if more than two people are fighting? Jiu Jitsu doesn't have an answer for multiple attackers. (Side note: As I said in a previous chapter, if there's more than one attacker, your chances of survival, no matter what you know, are diminished.) That being said, Jiu Jitsu has no answer at all for multiple attackers, which means that if there's more than one attacker, your chance of survival is zero. A well-known Jiu Jitsu practitioner by the name of Rener Gracie, who I respect and have taken workshops from, was once asked about multiple attackers. His answer was to run. Here's my problem with that: Your answer should always be to run if you have an opportunity to do so. Whether there is one attacker, two attackers, a guy with a knife, gun, or *whatever*, you should always run and get away before you choose to fight. Fighting should always be your last option. But we learn self-protection for that time when running is not an option.

There also aren't many strikes in Jiu Jitsu. Most Jiu Jitsu practitioners that I meet today would lose their shit if they were struck by a punch. The original form of Jiu Jitsu, however, was made to shut down strikes. But most schools that you find today have migrated toward the sports side of Jiu Jitsu and their training practices make strikes obsolete.

Punch a black belt in the face, he becomes a brown belt. Punch him again, purple. — Carlson Gracie

The other issue with Jiu Jitsu is that it takes a long time to become proficient. The average Jiu Jitsu practitioner trains as many as five times a week and still will not earn a blue or purple belt (Joe Rogan's assassin level) for a few years. The average person, especially in today's world, quite frankly, does not have or at least won't commit that kind of time.

All that being said, I still concur with Joe Rogan's assassin analogy. I do not think that anyone training to defend themselves should go without having at least a general knowledge of Jiu Jitsu in their repertoire. It is proven. It is effective. If you don't believe that it works, stop by your local Jiu Jitsu Dojo and have a few rolls.

A black belt only covers two inches of your ass. You have to cover the rest. — Royce Gracie

Taekwondo

Taekwondo is a Korean martial art characterized by punching and kicking techniques, with an emphasis on high head kicks, jumping spin kicks, and fast kicking techniques. The literal translation for Taekwondo is *kicking, punching, and the art of way.* This is the kind of martial art in which one attacks or defends with his or her hands and feet anytime or anywhere, with the occasional use of weapons.

As I said before, there are several different fighting arts/martial arts/self-protection systems out there. I will always contest that it is more about the mindset and the instructor, or the mindset of the instructor, than the actual art itself. For example, I received my Taekwondo black belt from an instructor by the name of Awesome Gerald

Dawson. The late Gerald Dawson was from the streets of Baltimore, again, during the '70s and '80s. At that time, he was a 250-to-300-pound fighter who took up Taekwondo so that he could better defend himself in the streets of Baltimore. He taught Taekwondo in the context of fighting. Although he did teach forms and traditional weapons and movements, his emphasis was always on the fight. He always said *"Don't be a pad killer"*, meaning someone good at hitting pads but terrible in an actual fight.

Taekwondo is a martial art and self-protection system in itself. I emphasize martial arts because Taekwondo's emphasis is based more on your character than your physical abilities. Every Taekwondo class starts the same way: you have to know the tenets of the system. Those include courtesy, integrity, perseverance, indomitable spirit, and self-control. The tenets of Taekwondo are drilled into the psyche of the students like fall breaks are drilled into the psyche of an Aikido or Judo practitioner. You don't go forward until you learn and embody the tenets. There is a deep and long history when it comes to the art of Taekwondo. Korean martial arts in general have a deep-rooted history and culture. I'll try not to get too much into the history and stick with more of the subject at hand, which is self-protection. That being said, you do need to know the history of this art to understand how Taekwondo applies and can be used in a self-protection situation.

There are many fighting styles that the Koreans used in the early to mid-1900s. In the 1900s, Gen. Choi Hong-hi created what we know today as Taekwondo. This system became the official fighting system for the South Korean military. Taekwondo is known for its kicking, speed, and power. Contrary to popular opinion, Taekwondo has a large variety of punches and hand strikes as well. One of Taekwondo's fighting philosophies is to be loose and light on your feet so you can react and create more speed. The idea is that the faster you are, the more powerful you are. This is why Taekwondo practitioners tend to stand straight more, at least while fighting, which is a lot different from other fighting styles such as Karate, wrestling, and Judo.

Taekwondo quickly became more of a sport than a fighting system. In the year 2000, it became an official sport of the Olympics. Today, Taekwondo is mostly practiced as a sport and a training system for kids and seniors.

But can they fight?

There have been several Taekwondo practitioners who have entered into MMA, or Mixed Martial Arts, which is now considered the proving grounds for effective fighting systems, and those who have done well. They include Anthony Pettis, Rose Namajunas, and Valentina Shevchenko, just to name a few. All of these practitioners got their roots from training in Taekwondo. But we don't even have to go that high up the totem pole. The punch that knocks you out is the punch you didn't see coming. That is true with kicks, takedowns, or anything else for that matter. Taekwondo focuses on speed and power. When I trained in Taekwondo, my instructors emphasized getting from where you are, point A, to where they are, point B, as fast as possible. It was called the blitz attack. *Strike first, strike hard,* Cobra Kai's Master Crease would say. Of course, he added no mercy, but we are talking about self-protection :). The average bad guy on the streets cannot defend against a decent Taekwondo kicker. Taekwondo works well for women because women generally have strong legs and are more flexible than men. Taekwondo has a big focus on confidence and character building. A trained Taekwondo practitioner carries themselves with a strong sense of pride and respect like a soldier in uniform. I cannot emphasize this enough. Carrying yourself with a certain amount of confidence helps you to avoid confrontations altogether, which is the best form of self-protection.

Pros

Although Taekwondo probably gets the most pushback and controversy when it comes to its effectiveness in self-protection, there are many pros to learning Taekwondo as a form of self-protection. One of the biggest pros of Taekwondo is that it increases your reaction time. You spend a lot of time developing speed. Not only does that increase your power, but it enables you to quickly be able to counter an incoming attack. This is a huge asset in a sudden violent situation. The hand strikes of a Taekwondo practitioner could be lethal if trained properly. One of these strikes is the arc-hand strike to the throat. The palm heel and hammer fist strike to the jaw area are also examples of how you can take out your assailant quickly.

The cons

In my experience, the controversy and pushback that Taekwondo gets as a whole are, I'm sad to say, legitimate. The system places a lot of emphasis on kicks, which would not be effective in close quarters. You also spend a lot of time learning forms and stances that will not be useful in an actual attack. Taekwondo is also primarily trained as a sport, which wouldn't be so bad if the sport replicated a real situation, but there are only a small number of situations in which a Taekwondo practitioner would have the room and space to execute those strategies.

All in all, I still feel that Taekwondo, barring you have the right instructor, is an excellent base for self-protection training. It's especially good for kids and young teenagers. If you've ever been kicked by a half-decent Taekwondo practitioner, which I have, you would agree.

When you get into Taekwondo, it teaches you the life skills of respect, self-control, and discipline—that's why I love it. I really attribute those skills to getting over my dad's death. If I didn't have that, I would have lost it. —Anthony Pettis, Former UFC Taekwondo Champion.

Boxing

Boxing is a combat sport in which two people, usually wearing protective gloves and other protective equipment, such as hand wraps and mouthpieces, throw punches at each other for a predetermined amount of time in a boxing ring.

So, if that is the case, why am I talking about boxing as it pertains to self-protection? Boxing has always been the go-to fighting system or self-protection system for any inner-city neighborhood. A large percentage of the young men who walk into a boxing gym are not looking to be the next heavyweight champion (perhaps the next Floyd Mayweather with all the glitz and glamor). The average young man walking into a boxing gym for the first time is looking to learn how to defend himself.

For example, there was a young twelve-year-old who walked into a boxing gym after having his bike stolen and said he wanted to learn how to fight so that he could beat the guy up. The young guy's name was Cassius Clay, later to be named Muhammed Ali, the greatest of all time. When I was growing up as a child and teenager, everyone wanted to learn to box. The boxers were the known tough guys of the neighborhood. Everyone would walk around sporting the neighborhood's boxing apparel on their backs. However, you had better not sport the apparel if you weren't part of the gym. One thing about inner-city kids, African-Americans in particular, is that at some point, you are taught how to throw a jab (left straight punch if you're right-handed), a cross (right straight punch), a hook (short range punch that travels across) and an uppercut (short range punch that travels up). The jab, cross, hook, and uppercut are the four strikes of the boxer. There are only four. Now, there are countless ways of throwing those four strikes, but there are only four strikes. Boxers are known for not only their toughness but also their conditioning. When you imagine the body of a boxer, you think of a perfectly sculptured specimen of a man, or in recent years, also of a woman, although many boxers nowadays may not fit that bill. There are two things that every decent boxer knows how to do: Number one, give a punch, and number two, take a punch. You will never meet a boxer that hasn't landed a punch or taken a punch during their training. Boxers are masters of timing, distance, footwork, and coordination. Most good boxing gyms are located in pretty rough areas, so a boxer's awareness and toughness come along with the package. There is also a lot of discipline that comes with being able to box. The discipline that a boxer must demonstrate in training helps to take the emotion out of the fight so that they can keep a level head. Boxing is often the number one self-protection and fighting system used by African-Americans all over the country.

But does it work in the street?

I don't think there is really or should be a debate about whether or not boxing would work in an actual situation. I don't think anybody would question whether Mike Tyson, Roberto Duran, or Jack Dempsey would be able to defend themselves in real situations. However, we don't have to go that high up the totem pole. If you find any amateur fighter who has had at least a year or two of boxing training, they're probably known for being one of the toughest and most respected guys in the neighborhood. Just like anything, though, there are pros and cons.

The pros

Boxers are experts at midrange and close-range fighting. Most planned and unplanned violent encounters take place in the midrange to close range proximity. Boxing, or at least some form of boxing, is the only system out of the four that we talk about in this book where getting punched is a normal part of training. Just like how a Jiu Jitsu practitioner knows he can do a rear naked choke or arm bar, a boxer knows he can punch you in the face and take a punch to the face. By the way, punching someone in the face is not as easy as you think.

The first time I went to a gun range, I remember putting the target far down the lane and firing my weapon. When I brought the target closer to me, I realized I hadn't hit the target at all. I had to put the target probably around six feet away from me to hit it, and even then, it wasn't a bull's-eye. It looked easy. It seemed easy, but when it came down to it, well, let's just say my weapons weren't calibrated. A boxer's weapons are always calibrated. Striking accuracy is a key ingredient for a boxer. Footwork is also a huge asset to a boxer in a self-protection situation. I teach my students that footwork makes the dream work. Being able to move in and out of the fight and knowing the distance in which you can hit or get hit could be the key to neutralizing your opponent. Footwork is also important when it comes to multiple attackers. The last thing you want to do with more than one opponent is to plant your feet and stand still. You have to be able to move. No one moves better than a boxer. The fitness of a boxer also plays a big part in boxers' being able to defend themselves. Just the way a boxer is built, with broad shoulders, biceps, and tree trunk legs, is enough to make an attacker choose someone else. The final pro to being a boxer in a self-protection situation is confidence. When you have trained repeatedly with other trained fighters, you feel a lot more confident going against an untrained opponent. Boxers train at full force and speed. It is what they do. Training at full force and speed gives you confidence. The more confidence you have, the less likely you are to use self-protection in the first place.

Everybody has a plan until they've been punched in the face. —Mike Tyson.

The cons

There has been a lot of debate in the last ten to twenty years about whether boxing is a complete self-protection system. That is mainly because of the popularity of MMA and Jiu Jitsu. Boxers have no training on what to do if the fight goes to the ground. Boxers also have no experience in using their legs as weapons. Not only do they not know how to kick or knee, but they also don't know how to defend against kicks or knees. In today's world, that leaves them open and vulnerable to a lot of would-be attackers. Another potential con when it comes to learning boxing for self-protection is the amount of potential damage that you could obtain during training. Unlike Jiu Jitsu, training at full force and speed, or sometimes even half speed, in a boxing gym requires that you get hit a lot. This is considered part of the sport and what needs to happen to move up the rankings of the boxing ladder. People who come in to learn to protect themselves are not thinking about progressing through the ranks of the sport. They just want to learn how to defend themselves. Risking the injuries that boxing can cause may not be worth it for the average person whose main motive is to just learn how to defend himself. As a matter of fact, after traveling through the environment that most boxing gyms are located in; seeing how hard boxers train and spar; and discovering what it takes for a boxer to get even half decent in their art, the average person just looking to take self-protection classes would say, "Why even bother?"

Boxing, as I mentioned earlier, has always been, and possibly always will be, the go-to fighting system of the African-American community. Martial arts are defined as the way a group of people defends themselves. Therefore, boxing is our martial art, and we've been defending our-selves well for quite some time. So yes, it works.

All power to the people! —The Black Panther Party

Krav Maga

Krav Maga is a military self-protection and fighting sys-tem developed for the Israel Defense Forces and Israeli security forces. It is derived from a combination of tech-niques sourced from boxing, wrestling, Judo, Aikido, and Karate. Krav Maga is known for its focus on real-world situations and its extreme efficiency. It is derived from the street fighting experience of Hungarian military martial artist Imi Lichtenfeld, who used his training as a boxer and wrestler while defending the Jewish quarter against fascist groups in Czechoslovakia during the mid to late 1930s. In the late 1940s, after he immigrated to Palestine, to what is now Israel, he began to provide lessons in combat training for what has become Krav Maga, the official training and combat system for the IDF (Israel Defense Forces).

I remember first hearing about Krav Maga back in the late 1990s. I had stopped doing martial arts for quite some time, and I was looking to get back into it. At the time, I was trying to decide which art I would study. I came across an article about which martial arts systems or self-protection systems were the most effective in the street. Krav Maga was number one. I thought to myself, *Well I will probably never be able to learn Krav Maga because it is in Israel*, but reading about the concepts intrigued me.

Years later, after leaving one of my training sessions at my Taekwondo school, I stumbled upon a Krav Maga school. I remembered saying, "Oh wow, I read about that some years ago. Let me go check it out." Honestly, when I first walked into the school, I didn't know much about Krav Maga. What I knew most about it was that Krav Maga schools mostly trained adults. At the time, I was tired of teaching only kids and I wanted to train and teach adults. After finally finding the right school for me, I quickly fell in love with the training philosophy, principles, and concepts, including the method by which Krav Maga is taught.

Krav Maga is based on principles. *Techniques will get you killed; principles will save your life:* Tim Larkin, When Violence is the Answer. When I read that, it only made me more confident in the teachings of Krav Maga. Those principles are as follows: Address the immediate danger; defend and counter-attack simultaneously; one defense must work against a variety of attacks; movements should be based on instincts; techniques must be assessable to the average person, not just athletes; training must be done from positions of disadvantage; training must include stress and experience of real attacks; and so on. Another reason why I fell so deep into Krav Maga is its simplicity. I don't like to think much. If it doesn't come naturally to me, I don't want to do it. Krav Maga's biggest principles are movements and techniques that must be easy to learn. The book, *Complete Krav Maga* by Darren Levine, founder of Krav Maga Worldwide, tells a story about Imi visiting him in the summer of 1982 in Los Angeles.

When Imi came to visit me, I had just bought a new sports car, and I was really excited to show it to him. I was really proud of that car. When Imi got in the car, he started shifting and fidgeting around, reaching over his shoulder. He looked unhappy. Finally, I asked him what was wrong. He said, "This car is not good. The seatbelt is too far back. I can't reach it with my right hand. I can't reach it with my left hand. I'm a lazy one. It needs to be easy, or people won't wear their seatbelts. It's not safe". At the time, Darren was disappointed. *I wanted him to be impressed with my car,* he said. *But later, I realized that he looked at the seat belt the same way he looked at everything. It had to be simple and effective or people wouldn't be able to do it. That was Krav Maga.*

Krav Maga has also come under a lot of scrutiny for several reasons. Some are legit, and some are not so legit. One of the reasons that people attack Krav Maga so much is that they don't understand it. They watch videos on YouTube and see the mediocre techniques and say, "Well, that's way too simple" or "It would never work in a real situation." What they don't understand is that the movements and techniques that are taught in Krav Maga are taught to back up the principles of Krav Maga. As explained in *Complete Krav Maga, we must start with actual techniques. If we give students abstract principles, they will have nowhere to begin their training. This would be like plucking the strings of the guitar, describing music theory, then handing the instrument to a new student and asking him to figure out the song for himself. He would feel lost. Instead, we teach him notes. We help build simple songs and chords, and soon he understands that the variations of the notes and chords are nearly limitless.* This philosophy and principles are really what made me fall for Krav Maga. It is also what has attracted Krav Maga to so many people. As I said before, people nowadays want things that are fast and easy.

But does it work?

I find it hard to believe or understand when people question whether or not a combat system used by an entire group of people is effective, especially when it comes to something like a military-based system. If the military were to devise an ineffective system, that military would crumble in battle. If anyone knows anything about the Israeli mindset, they know that the Israelis believed that if they were to lose a war, they would also lose their country. So, when they fought, they fought relentlessly. Their motto was *I win or I die.* No military force or group of people with that principle or mindset would use a system if it wasn't effective. But like anything, there are pros and cons.

The pros

The pros of Krav Maga are undoubtedly its training methods and ideology. It's all about the drills. I believe in the 'training slow is training fast theory,' but I also know that to be able to perform a technique, you have to put yourself under the same or close to the same amount of stress that you will be under on the game day. Krav Maga has countless drills that are created for just that reason. They have also created drills that they can do at full speed, just like Jiu Jitsu, without injuring the practitioners. After all, what good would an army be if most of the soldiers were injured when it was time to do battle? Krav Maga teaches you to handle a variety of common real-life situations and violent encounters. They teach you to punch just like the boxers. They teach you to kick just like the Taekwondo practitioners. They teach you to grapple like a Jiu Jitsu practitioner. They teach you to deal with weapons or fight against common weapons like knives, sticks, gun threats, etc. Anything can happen if you are caught behind enemy lines and you can't get to your weapon. Because of the variety of training, a good Krav Maga practitioner is well prepared for a wide variety of scenarios. It's also a great training system for those who are not as athletic, big, or strong as their adversaries. Remember that when Krav Maga was created, a war was going on in which the soldiers were of all weight sizes and athletic abilities. The system had to work for everyone. People who may not have the physical attributes to become an MMA fighter can still be proficient at Krav Maga.

The cons

'Jack of all trades, master of none.' Krav Maga practitioners Box but Krav Maga practitioners aren't great boxers. Krav Maga practitioners kick, but Krav Maga practitioners aren't great kickers. Krav Maga practitioners grapple, but if a Krav Maga practitioner was to go on to the ground with a Jiu Jitsu practitioner, the outcome would favor the Jiu Jitsu practitioner. Krav Maga focuses on being able to learn the system quickly; the average Krav Maga practitioner trains twice a week. The average boxer, Jiu Jitsu player, and even Taekwondo fighter trains for five, maybe even six days a week. I don't care what you do. Two days a week will not make you as proficient as someone who trains for five. The popularity of Krav Maga has made it more commercialized. Finding a legitimate Krav Maga school is like finding a company to invest in that will become the next Google. It's also difficult to find instructors that actually know Krav Maga and understand its principles and know how to teach them properly.

Fortunately for the average Krav Maga practitioner, their goal is not to learn to defend themselves against a black belt Jiu Jitsu practitioner, a world champion boxer, or the next Jhoon Rhee. A Krav Maga practitioner's goal is to be able to quickly defend themselves against an average attacker, get away quickly, and go home safe. You don't have to train five days a week for five years to do that. What you need is a warrior mindset, the willingness to learn and train, and a fighting spirit. That is also Krav Maga.

"People respect power, and it comes in many forms. Krav Maga is power, and people will respect you for knowing it."
Imi Lichtenfeld

Others:

Originally, I was only going to include the arts/self-defense systems that I have studied and trained in, but I have decided to also include a few others that I feel are effective. Although I have little or no experience in these other systems, as I will explain later, you don't need direct experience to be able to transfer knowledge. What you need is research. Here's what I found over the years about these other systems.

Judo

Judo is a modern Japanese form of unarmed combat. It was created by Jigoro Kano as a martial art focused on free sparring instead of pre-arranged forms. It emphasizes throws. However, they also include pins, takedowns, joint locks, chokes, and falls.

Pros

The Judo practitioner is very proficient as it pertains to close-quarter combat. They are masters at getting their opponents off balance and pinning them to the ground.

Cons

They do not fend while up against multiple opponents. It's also difficult for smaller opponents to deal with larger ones. This is why Gracie modified the system and created BJJ.

Wrestling

Wrestling is one of the oldest forms of unarmed combat. *There are also many different forms of wrestling.* It's defined as a combat sport involving grappling-type techniques such as clinch fighting, throws and takedowns, joint locks, pins, and other grappling holds. Wrestling, like boxing and now even Jiu Jitsu, is mostly looked at as a sport. However, just like boxing, I've included it here as a self-defense system because a half-decent wrestler could pretty much rag doll the average person their size if they got a hold of them.

Pros

The wrestler has the following advantages:

- Great at close-quarter fighting

- Unmatched conditioning

- Great at fighting on the ground

- Relentless fighting spirit

Cons

- They're not good at throwing or defending against strikes (The old saying is: who would win against a boxer and a wrestler? The one that gets off first).

- They have no defense against common weapons.

- They have no defense against multiple opponents.

- It is not conducive for a smaller person that is going up against a larger attacker.

Muay Thai

Muay Thai, as defined, is a martial art and combat system also known as Thai Boxing that uses stand-up striking along with various clinching techniques. This discipline is known as the "art of eight limbs." Two fists, two elbows, two knees, and two shins. However, they also use their feet as well. Muay Thai has become very popular among MMA fighters. When you see an MMA training center, two things that they will almost always include are Jiu Jitsu and Muay Thai.

Pros

Muay Thai practitioners

- Have powerful strikes;

- Have experience in defending and taking strikes; and

- Are very good mid-to-close range fighters.

Cons

- No ground fighting experience

- No experience against common weapons

Chapter Eight

The Instructors

Those That Can

Myth: A good instructor has a lot of direct, real-world experience in what they are teaching.

I started training fighters when I was about fourteen years old in my grandmother's garage in my old neighborhood. Sometimes, my play brother would stop by to help. He sometimes wore a Band-Aid over his eye. The crazy thing was that he hadn't been in a fight. He wore it to look tough so people would think he knew what he was talking about. He didn't, but it worked. It made it look like he had been in a real fight. One of the techniques Krav Maga is known for is the system's handgun takeaways. I have personally met over a hundred instructors who teach handgun takeaways, but I have only met three who have ever had to do a handgun takeaway in a real situation.

I have also gone to countless active shooter seminars taught by a variety of instructors, but I have never met an instructor — or any person, for that matter — who has ever had the horrific experience of being in an actual active shooter situation.

I have met hundreds of instructors who teach how to escape a two-handed front choke, but not many, including myself, have ever had anyone attempt to attack them with a two-handed front choke. So, does that mean that these people are not real self-protection instructors? Of course, it doesn't. Going through or being involved with those specific experiences does not qualify someone to teach another person or group of people how to deal with those situations.

I often read the comments people leave on self-protection instructional videos, and I see the same pattern: more often than not, people comment on the attacker, not on the actual defense. Comments are almost always negative and focus on how the attacker in the video is being nonresistant. "Anybody can do that defense if you just stand there." "No one actually attacks like that." "How about you try that when someone is trying to fight you back?" These are all comments that I have heard or read in the dreaded comment section of an instructional video. I noticed that these kinds of comments mostly pertain to self-protection instructional videos. When you see a Jiu Jitsu demonstration and the black belt instructor is teaching you how to do an arm-bar or an Americana, you never get comments on why their demo partner isn't resisting. When you see a boxing coach giving a demonstration on a boxer who is standing still, you never get comments about how a hook wouldn't work if the guy just ducked. The same with MMA. After some thought, I realized that the reason why you get those comments on self-protection instruction is that people know that Jiu Jitsu fighters have experience doing Jiu Jitsu. Boxing coaches actually have boxing experience. MMA coaches have experience in the cage. Self-protection instructors, on the other hand, don't always have any experience when it comes down to what they are instructing. That makes them a target. That puts them under the radar. That means that everything they do, people will question. I get it. I understand. That being said, people with experience are not always the best instructors. The world of sports offers some great examples of what I'm talking about. There are numerous examples of experienced, legendary players who later went on to become not-so-great coaches. Magic Johnson, often regarded as the greatest point guard of all time, coached a team for one season and led them to a ten-game losing streak. The great Wayne Gretzky, arguably the greatest and most experienced hockey player of all time, was a horrible coach. Isaiah Thomas and Rampage Jackson are other examples and the list goes on. On the other hand, some of the greatest boxing trainers, NBA, and NFL coaches were not great players at all. Phil Jackson, who coached Michael Jordan and Kobe Bryant, and Bill Belichick, one of the winningest coaches in the NFL, are perfect examples. Hell, for that matter, some have never played. Going through or being involved with those specific experiences does not qualify someone to teach another person or group of people how to deal with those situations.

Myth: Where you're from makes you a good instructor.

If you are from Brazil, that must mean that you are an excellent Jiu Jitsu instructor. It's called Brazilian Jiu Jitsu, for God's sake. If you are Korean, that must mean that you are an excellent instructor in teaching someone to do jump spinning heel kicks. Isn't that what Koreans do? If you're a brother from the projects, that must mean you can fight. I mean, don't all black guys know how to fight? Oh, and here's the best one of them all: Everyone from Israel knows Krav Maga, the whole country. When you think about them, these stereotypes are quite funny.

Myth: Your occupation makes you a good instructor.

If you're a police officer, well, that must mean you have experience, and therefore you should be able to teach. The truth is that the majority of police officers have virtually no hand-to-hand combat experience. The lack of training because the police department doesn't pay for them is quite a shame. I have trained countless police officers as well as civilians, and trust me when I tell you that the civilians are not only in better shape but better all-around fighters. Most police officers have no idea what to do without their guns. I know this because the police officers that train and know what to do have told me so.

How about the military? If you have been in the military, that must mean that you are a good instructor and have a lot of experience. I honor my fellow Americans who are willing to put their lives on the line to defend this great country that we live in. That being said, being in the military does not qualify you to be a good self-protection instructor. Most military people that you will meet, at least nowadays, have never even seen battle. Let's hope it stays that way.

What if they are bouncer security at a tough nightclub or bar? I'm sure they have seen some action. I agree. I think that if you have worked security at a tough nightclub, chances are you have been in a few scrapes. I also know people who have owned several cars in their lifetime, but I would never get them to teach my child how to drive one.

Myth: Someone with a lot of trophies, who has won championships, is a good instructor.

Surely, someone who has dozens of trophies in their window is a good instructor. Don't be so sure. I know this is hard for many to read, but there are a lot of martial arts instructors who open schools and then create a window display of trophies they have purchased to make their school or themselves look more reputable. I'm not saying it happens all the time, but it is important to know that a trophy can be purchased at any local trophy shop. It's not like the trophy shop asks you for credentials, either. I remember going to a trophy shop for the first time to purchase a plaque for one of my students. The owner of the shop asked, "Why not just get her a trophy?" I had always assumed that you had to be part of an organization to purchase a trophy. How naive. But let's give them the benefit of the doubt. Let's assume that the trophies are real. My next question would be, "Who does the trophy belong to?" Has the instructor been in several tournaments and do the trophies belong to him? If so, that makes that person a good fighter or competitor, but it doesn't necessarily mean they are a good instructor. Do the trophies belong to students? If so, why don't the students keep the trophy? I had an instructor that made it mandatory for his students to donate all first-place trophies to the school so that others would be able to see the trophy in the window. My next question is, what is the trophy for? Does the instructor have several grand champions as students? Is the school known for winning first place every year in the All Valley High Championship? The problem is, they don't give out trophies for surviving an actual sudden violent attack. So, having a multitude of trophies does not make you a proficient self-protection instructor.

Myth: All great self-protection instructors have impressive resumes.

Self-protection instructors spend a lot of time building up their resumes. It's good marketing. After all, we have businesses to run. Sometimes, students actually prefer impressive resumes over good instruction. Maybe an instructor has a lot of followers on their YouTube channel. Perhaps they've been featured in a few magazines or news broadcasts. Perhaps they have documented 'over thirty years of experience'. Just writing this book and being able to add 'author of' to my list of accomplishments is going to beef up my instructor résumé. Full disclosure: writing this book does not make me a good instructor. There are many more ingredients to the recipe. I would argue that none of the above is even the main ingredient. So, what is?

Before I dive into the qualities of a good instructor, I want you to know that I'm speaking from experience. You see, I once trained for about six months with a gentleman who I won't name but who told me that he was a nationally known sports Karate champion. He told me he had a system that could not be beaten. At the time, I was very interested in being a sports Karate fighter, which I became later on, and this particular "instructor" was the first guy that I came across. I trained with this brother every day for months on end, only to find out later that he was far from a great fighting instructor. Not only was he not a national champion himself, he had not trained any champions either. The things that he taught me were, as I know now, laughable at best. How was I supposed to know? I had never fought in a Karate tournament. I didn't know any sports Karate fighters. The most I knew about a good instructor was *wax on, wax off*. Unfortunately, that wasn't the first time I experienced a subpar instructor, and it wasn't the last. I definitely went through the school of hard knocks when it came to finding the right instructors or instruction. The good news is that I can now tell you how to not make the same mistakes I made when looking for an instructor and I can steer you in the right direction.

Those that teach

Fact: A good instructor has mastered the art of teaching.

A good instructor can teach an effective technique proficiently. I recently read an article that stated great coaches know the common points of their trade. They know which words, plans, plays, and strategies are most effective at clearing up confusion and which methods are the best to be implemented. It all comes down to character and execution, not skill. This is not only true for a great coach, but for a good practitioner as well. I think that article does a fantastic job of explaining what a good coach or instructor is. Albert Einstein said, "If you can't <u>explain</u> it simply, you don't understand it well enough." I disagree. Many people are very good at doing things. They understand what they're doing, but they have a difficult time explaining it. Knowing how to properly articulate a particular technique or principle is a skill that you are not necessarily born with. It is something that has to be taught to you. I can stand up in front of a class of students and throw kicks, punches, and knees all day long, but if I can't clearly explain to my students how to do these maneuvers themselves, what's the point?

I'll give you another example from personal experience: During a firearms class I once participated in, the instructor told me all of the tests he had to pass to become a certified firearms instructor, including shooting drills, safety requirements, and several written exams. This was all about being an expert marksman and knowing your way around a firearm. Never did he mention taking a class on how to teach someone to shoot the damn thing. As good as he was as a shooter, his class was terrible. I later took firearm lessons from a colleague of mine who was also a school teacher, and I walked away feeling much more confident and informed in my ability to shoot a firearm. The school teacher knew how to teach.

Fact: A good instructor has good character.

You have to be able to master your emotions to be a good instructor. The last thing I would want is an emotional Jiu Jitsu instructor, who argued with his wife just before class, teaching me how to do an ankle lock. Good character goes a long way when it comes to being a good instructor. One of the things I look for in the students I recruit to become instructors has always been good character. A person of good character chooses to do the right thing because he or she believes it is morally right to do so. An instructor with good character would not knowingly teach a technique that they did not feel would work. An instructor with good character would not teach or attempt to teach an effective technique if they did not feel that they could do so proficiently. An instructor with good character would seek the proper training to transfer the proper knowledge properly. An instructor with good character cares about their students and generally wants them to learn.

Fact: A good instructor invites questions from students.

They don't mind answering questions. Some instructors get offended when you ask them a question. There are schools where it is considered rude to question the instructor. When asked a question, instead of explaining the reason behind the technique, the instructor defends the technique that they're teaching. Oftentimes, when instructors are offended by questions and defend their teaching rather than further explaining what they've just taught, it is because of their insecurity in either the technique or their ability to teach it. If that is the case, then that instructor has no business on the floor teaching that particular technique or principle. When it pertains to self-protection, you are responsible for instructing someone to do something that could save their life. That responsibility should not be taken lightly, and an instructor with good character would not do so.

SELF-DEFENSE WHY EVEN BOTHER?   79

Fact: A good instructor inspires their students to learn.

Another thing to look for in a good instructor is the ability to motivate and inspire you to learn. If you think back to when you were a child and you were first able to identify your favorite subject in grade school, that subject was often taught by your favorite teacher at the time. That particular subject, in most cases, becomes your favorite subject throughout your childhood or at least, until you choose another favorite teacher. Good teachers and instructors not only inspire you to learn but also make you feel good about being a student.

When I was in high school, I had a teacher by the name of Vincent Massey. Vincent Massey taught data processing at the Burdick training center in Washington, D.C. I had no interest at all in data processing. I took the class as an elective because I needed extra credits but there was something about the way Mr. Massey taught and carried himself. Unlike the other teachers, I felt as though he cared not just about teaching me data processing but about who I would become in life. I was far from an honor roll student and oftentimes, I wouldn't even show up for my other classes but trust me when I tell you, I never missed data processing. For a short time, I had decided that being a data processor was what I wanted to do for a living. I credit

Vincent Massey for helping me to become the man I am today. I haven't seen him for over thirty-five years, but if he's out there and if he's reading this book, I salute you. That is the effect that a good instructor should have on their student.

Fact: A good instructor is approachable.

A good instructor is thankful and approachable. The martial arts/self-protection world is packed with instructors with mega-sized egos. They teach in a way that would lead you to believe that it should be an honor for you to be a part of their class. I took a seminar from Rener Gracie, the grandson of Helio Gracie, the founder of Brazilian Jiu Jitsu. There were over 250 students in attendance, ranging from white to black belts. Rener Gracie is not only a high-level Jiu Jitsu instructor but is also a personality superstar. He has over 500,000 followers on his YouTube channel. After the seminar, Rener took pictures with every student that attended the workshop. Although he was late for an appointment and had taught Jiu Jitsu for six hours straight, I had a few questions that he didn't get a chance to answer during the session. He asked that I accompany him as he walked to his car, and he would try to answer a couple of questions on the way. I was one of the over 250 students who were in attendance, and somehow, he made me feel as if he was there solely for me. That is the trait of a good instructor. I've taken workshops from other high-level instructors in various arts. Some didn't speak to anyone beforehand and didn't speak to anyone afterward. They taught as if they were teaching from a throne. That is not a sign of a good instructor.

Fact: A good instructor will make you feel safe.

A good instructor, even though they are teaching something as scary as how to defend yourself against a person that may be trying to kill you, will make you feel safe while you're learning. Some instructors are intimidating. Some are intimidating on purpose. Perhaps they think if they look the part, you won't question what they are teaching. Intimidation is not an effective teaching method.

Fact: A great instructor will earn your trust.

I once had a boxing coach who was a very good boxer. He was even great at explaining it. But for some reason, I was very nervous about sparring with him. I would avoid him like I would avoid being in an elevator with three people without their masks during the COVID-19 pandemic. Even after sparing with him once or twice, I still didn't trust him. There was something about him that didn't make me feel safe. Later, I found that others felt the same way. You have to trust your instructor. Trust is earned, not given. A good instructor has a way of earning your trust. Great instructors will earn it rather quickly. Perhaps it's the way that they speak. Perhaps it's a well-timed joke. Perhaps it's their emphasis on safety in training. Whatever the method, every good instructor knows the importance of trust. They know that it's up to them to earn your trust, and they do what is necessary to accomplish it. As it is explained in my Krav Maga Instructor handbook, *"A student will feel you have the power to hurt them, but don't. You have the power to make them safer, and you do."*

When you know what to look for, identifying the traits of good instructors is not as hard as one may think. All you have to do is choose a reputable martial arts/self-protection system that suits your needs and then look for an instructor with the right character to correctly transfer the knowledge.

This is the first and last thing my students see when they enter and leave my training room.

Watch your Thoughts, For they become words.

Watch your Words, For they become Actions.

Watch your Actions, For they become Habits.

Watch your Habits, For they become Character.

Watch your Character, For it becomes your DES-TINY!

Character is one of the biggest requirements of a good instructor as well as a good student.

Chapter Nine

Female Self-protection Instructors

As we talk about what it takes to be a good instructor, it's also important to discuss female self-protection instructors.

Self-protection for women has become a hot commodity in the last ten to fifteen years. With more women coming in to take self-protection classes, there is also a need for more female self-protection instructors. The thought is that women are more comfortable training and learning from women. In some situations, that statement can be true. Women teaching other women self-protection is a good thing. Women teaching men self-protection is a GREAT thing. Let's talk about it.

Some years back, I got a call from a potential student who wanted to come in and take Krav Maga classes. He spoke highly of my videos and some of the things that he had read and heard about. I was happy to have him come in and try one of the classes, but right before I scheduled him, he wanted to know if CDK had any female self-defense instructors. He then asked, "Will they be teaching the class that I will be attending? I only asked because I don't want to take a self-protection class from a female. I don't think a female can teach men how to defend themselves." This simple question turned into a long conversation with the potential student as I went on to explain my opinion about female self-protection instructors.

There are a lot of men that feel this way about female instructors, so let me get straight to the point. In my opinion, which is derived from years of experience, women make better self-protection instructors than men. Here is why: A complete self-protection system should cover three things. First, how to deal with multiple attackers (when I speak of multiple attackers, I'm speaking of two or three at the most, not twelve). Second, how to deal with someone who has a weapon. Third, how to deal with someone bigger and stronger than you.

If your system does not cover at least two out of those three things, then your system, in my opinion, is not a complete self-protection system. One of those two things has to be dealing with an attacker that is bigger and stronger than you. If the person that you are defending yourself against does not have a friend and does not have a weapon, there's a high probability that he will be bigger and stronger than you. The average man is bigger and stronger than the average female, so the average female cannot rely on her size and strength to defend herself against the average male. She must use techniques that make her a more accurate practitioner and probably a better instructor.

In my journey, I have had only three female instructors. I know several female instructors, but I have only had three that have trained me. The first was an instructor named Sarah. Sarah was one of my favorite instructors. She taught with so much passion, so much meaning, and so much energy. I hired Sarah to help me prepare for my Level Four Krav Maga belt exam. At the time, we could not train at the school, so I invited Sarah to come over to my side of town. I trained at the weight lifting gym in Prince George's (PG) County, Maryland. PG County would be considered the rougher part of town as compared to the gentrified locations in Washington, D.C. Sarah caught the subway, came on over to the gym and began to train one of my partners and me. We used the aerobics room that was right beside the weightlifting area. The weight room was always packed and noisy. You could see into the aerobics room from the weight area. As Sarah taught, the weight room was completely silent. You could hear a pin drop. The reason? All of the brothers in the weight room stopped to watch Sarah teach us the techniques. That's how good and proficient she was as an instructor. To this day, when I run into some of the fellows from the old gym, the first thing they ask me is if I still train with that lady from the gym. Some even swear they have seen her on TV fighting in the UFC. Sarah has never fought in the UFC. However, she was that good.

My second female self-protection instructor's name is Kelly. Kelly is the highest-ranking female Krav Maga practitioner and instructor in our parent organization, Krav Maga Worldwide. Every instructor in our organization has trained under Kelly at some point in their career. When it comes to teaching or assisting with a technique, she is the most accurate instructor I have worked with in my entire thirty years of training. I am always amazed by her ability to pinpoint and correct an issue with my techniques. Kelly is responsible for teaching me how to teach. As stated earlier, passing information on to a person or group of people in the proper way is a skill. *"Skill can only be developed from hours and hours of beating on your craft.”* - Will Smith. Committing yourself to all those hours takes dedication. To become a great instructor, you must be dedicated. I have not met many self-protection instructors as dedicated as Kelly.

The third female instructor that I worked under, we will just call Sgt. Betty Badass. Sgt. Badass is the Krav Maga combat instructor for one of the largest sheriff's departments in the country. She is responsible for making sure that the cadets that come out of the department can defend themselves without their weapons. She is about 5 feet 2 inches and weighs under 115 pounds. I had the honor of briefly assisting her in one of her classes, and let me tell you—I have never seen a person that size command a room with that many men and get that much respect. These guys weren't exactly tiny. I was amazed at how she not only captured the trust and respect of the candidates, but I was also hugely impressed by the way she instructed them. I still use some of her teaching methods in my classes today.

If you want to be taught correctly, if you want to make sure that you are using a technique that does not require you to be bigger or stronger than your adversary, if you ever find a female who is teaching a reputable self-protection class, whether you're a woman or a man, my suggestion is that you put this book down right now and go take her class.

Chapter Ten

How to Train for Self-Protection

You have decided that you want to learn about self-protection. You've decided what system of the arts you want to study. You found the right instructor. Now comes the most important part: how to train for self-protection.

How to Train for Self-Defense was the original title for this book. It wasn't even supposed to be a book. It was just a blog. When I was sharing my ideas with a friend, he replied, "Wow! That's a lot. Why Even Bother?" And here we are. Self-protection training is a complex subject and falls under different opinions depending on what you're studying and who's teaching it. Before I go any further, let me say that if you have found a good instructor, he or she should know the best way to train for what he or she is teaching. What I am giving you here is general information on how to train, particularly in the world of self-protection/martial arts. I believe in principle-based training. So, what does principal-based training mean? A principle-based system or principle-based training means that your training will always fall back on certain rules and guidelines. For example, one of the principles of Jiu Jitsu training is energy efficiency. Every technique done under that system involves the mindset of not using more energy or strength than your opponent. One of the training principles of Taekwondo is perseverance. Every Taekwondo technique that you practice is exceptionally hard to get right, and you must persevere to learn it. You must also understand that, as a martial artist, you can never fully master a martial art. There's always something that can be improved, no matter how technical or flexible you are. Therefore, without the principle of perseverance in your training, you will not succeed. A principle of boxing is that when your opponent misses, you must make them pay. A good defense is only as valuable as the openings it creates. Of course, there's Krav Maga. Everything you learn must be easily applicable. You must be able to do the techniques under stress. You must attack by learning to block and counter simultaneously or immediately. These are training principles as they pertain to different arts. However, you should have a set of training principles that you follow in general. There are rules to the game, and contrary to what the saying says, rules are not made to be broken. Here are ten rules or commandments that I have formulated through my years of instructing and training. They are "The CDK ten commandments of training."

Commandment #1

Learn slow to go fast.

No skill in life can be learned by starting fast. Although this law or principle makes sense to everyone who hears it, it is a skill that is rarely practiced by young men. Young men come into the training center and it's almost always *go go go*, especially with my teen athletes. No matter if they are learning something as basic as a jab (straight left punch) or something as complex as a Jiu Jitsu triangle, you will be lucky to get three slow repetitions before they are moving at full speed. This is a huge flaw in their training. "*You fight a young man. Nothing held back. Admirable but mistaken*" —Bane, The Dark Knight Rises. To really embody a technique or movement, that technique or movement must be done and repeated at a slow pace. I often tell my students that they should train at the speed and level of their proficiency. If you are a batter on a baseball team and the pitcher throws the ball and you are missing most of your swings, the first thing that you should do is have the pitcher slow down the pitch. This will give you the ability to pinpoint where your problem lies. Once you have pinpointed the problem, you can start to work on it. As your accuracy increases with the slow pitches, the pitcher can then start increasing the speed. This, too, should be done slowly.

I often see professional baseball players throw the ball down the field so fast that it amazes me that the batter is ever able to hit one ball. In actuality, the batter does not see the ball coming as fast as I do. Depending on the pitcher, he doesn't see the ball coming fast at all. To prove this theory, baseball even has a pitch called the fastball. To me, all the pitches are fast. But not to someone who's practiced slowly and sped up over time. I don't play baseball. I am a fighter. However, the laws of training are the same and apply to everything in life, self-protection training included. If you want to have a bad day at the gym, learn how to block a punch for the first time. Pick the fastest puncher in the gym, and have them just throw punches at your face at full speed. Not a fun day. This is where you hear some people make the statement, "But in the street, they're not going to go slow. They're going to throw them fast." This may be true, but if you don't first learn to do things slowly, you will never be able to block fast anyway. Some trainers even believe in only training slowly, and that you will naturally speed up when it is necessary.

Training too fast is a problem that most young men have. However, it is not as big of a problem with females and older men. Females often train without their egos and have no problem slowing down their pace to learn properly. Older men were once young men who now realize the error in their ways. So, no matter what you are learning how to do, whether it's a punch, a block, a kick, a choke hold, or even just how to wrap your hands properly, learn your skill slowly and you will save yourself a lot of time in the long run.

Commandment #2

You must go fast.

Eventually, after repetitive slow training, you need to speed up. This is where my opinion differs from some other self-protection instructors. I believe that it is imperative that you train and learn at a slow pace, but I also believe that it is just as imperative that you pressure test your skills at a realistic pace. You need to pressure test your skills not only to improve them but also to build the confidence necessary to do them when you need them. I was watching the making of one of Beyoncé's concerts, and it was not only amazing but mind-opening. It was amazing how much work she put into her preparation and rehearsals. Of course, all of the early rehearsals started slowly. 1-2-3-4-5-6-7-8, 1-2-3-4-5-6-7-8. Every beat was counted out loud until everyone was in one accord. A few weeks away from the opening day, they started to not only increase the pace but also started to mimic exactly what it would be like on the day of the show. The lights, the cameras, and the action were all done exactly the way they would be done on stage. Timing is everything. "You've got to get the time right," she would say to the performers. If you've ever been to a Beyoncé concert, you know they are magnificent. Everyone is on point. Every explosion, every beat, and even the lights are done with precision and on time. I do not believe that this would be possible without dress rehearsals done in real time. You first have to go slowly, but you must eventually go fast.

My instructor would always tell me that fighting is about timing and distance. You cannot learn timing without moving at real speed. I learned this the hard way when I was training for my 2nd Dan black belt in Krav Maga. My strategy was to train and practice all of my techniques at a slow pace, assuming that I would naturally or automatically be able to increase my pace on test day. My reason for doing so was not only to perfect my techniques. Training at a slower pace also decreased the chances of getting injured before the test. The 2nd Dan black belt test only happens once a year and if you miss it, you have to wait a whole year to take another test. Of course, I would do my conditioning workouts to make sure that I was in great shape, but I would do that separately. All the technical training was slow. That was my first time going into a test without the utmost confidence. I knew that I could do all the techniques, but what would happen — or what was going to happen — when I had to do them at full speed and under stress remained a mystery. The test was four days long, and by the third day, I knew that I had made a huge mistake in my preparation. What I noticed most was that my timing was way off. When someone is swinging punches, sticks, and kicks at you, timing is a pretty important thing to have. *"If you can do it slowly, you can do it fast. If you're doing it fast, that doesn't mean you're doing it right."* That's what I used to say to my students before my 2nd Dan black belt failed attempt. The next year, I changed my strategy. I took the Beyoncé concert prep strategy. I started training slowly at the beginning and a few weeks before showtime I trained at a pace. After passing my test, I changed my quote to: *"You go slow first and go fast last. But you must go fast!"*

Commandment #3

Patience

When I looked up the word *patience*, I found several definitions. They were so relevant to the subject at hand that I couldn't just give you one. So here are three:

Patience: the capacity to accept or tolerate delay, trouble, or suffering without getting angry or upset.

Patience: the ability to wait, or to continue doing something despite difficulties, or to suffer without complaining or being annoyed.

Patience: the ability to endure difficult circumstances.

Patience involves present perseverance and tolerance of provocation without responding with disrespect/anger, especially when faced with long-term difficulties or being able to wait for a long period without getting irritated or bored. It is also used to refer to the character trait of being steadfast. There goes that character thing again.

Patience is a mandatory ingredient to becoming a proficient martial artist. After all, Rome was not built in a day. I often have new students come in and one of the first questions that they ask is how long it will take them to get to either the next level or a black belt in Krav Maga.

Krav Maga was developed to quickly prepare the Israeli military soldiers for battle. Part of the allure of Krav Maga is that it doesn't take a long time to learn. The fact that it doesn't take a long time to learn does not mean that you will become a black belt on your first day of training. Just like with anything in life, the good things take time. Time is not something that people tend to cherish nowadays. Everybody wants it and everybody wants it now. The old saying "patience is a virtue" is a phrase that seems to be fading out of our culture. You must put in the time. Jiu Jitsu has taught me the art of patience more so than any other fighting system that I have trained in or studied. The techniques are complicated. The classes are slow-paced and you lose a lot more than you win when it pertains to sparring and training. That would probably explain the high dropout rate of beginner white and blue belts that start training in Jiu Jitsu. That would also explain the high level of proficiency of the upper belts. They are the ones who stuck it out. They are the ones who stayed in the game, persevered, and showed the virtue of patience. In a self-protection scenario, they are the ones who could kill you or give you serious bodily injury if they were forced to defend themselves. I often tell newer students not to concentrate on how soon or how fast they will get to the next level. It is more proficient to focus on getting better at what you are learning today.

"You don't set out to build a wall. You don't start by saying, 'I'm going to build the biggest, baddest wall that's ever been built.' You don't start there. You say 'I'm going to lay this brick as perfectly as a brick can be laid.' If you do that every single day, soon you will have a wall." — Will Smith.

Learning to defend yourself is no different than building a wall that is built one brick at a time. Self-protection is learned one class at a time. Every time you lay a brick, the wall is closer to being built. Every time you take a class, workshop, or practice, you are becoming more proficient at knowing how to defend yourself. First, you must start, and then you must stay the course. *Wax on, wax off. Patience, Danielson.*

Commandment #4

Conditioning beats class.

A few years ago, I had the honor of being able to train in Israel with a few of the all-stars of Krav Maga. One of them was Ran Nakash. Ran is one of the former commanders of the Krav Maga division in the Israeli Military. He teaches Krav Maga, boxing, and other various fighting systems at his boxing gym, called Nakash Boxing. When you walk into the gym, the first thing you see painted high in yellow on a brick wall is the phrase *Conditioning*

Beats Class. After training with Ran for just an hour or so, you quickly understand the meaning of the sign. Just like the famous quote by Vince Lombardi, "Fatigue makes cowards of us all," Ran used words in this context to stress the importance of conditioning, both mental and physical, whether it is in facing a battle or stepping onto a football field. All of the fighters who trained at Nakash Boxing were in exceptionally great shape. I remember thinking to myself that if any mega promoter went to Israel, they would definitely find champions.

When you are under attack, you will be put under extreme pressure. When you are put under pressure, you are placed in a highly stressful circumstance. I have read that the average street fight lasts forty-seven seconds. Even for a person who is well trained, forty-seven seconds can feel like forty-seven minutes. If you are not in the right condition to last for the entire fight, then it doesn't make a difference how many techniques you know or how good you are at them, because you won't be able to perform them. *Conditioning beats class, and fatigue makes cowards of us all.*

I recently watched a devastating video in which a man was stabbed repeatedly in the back by a bad guy with a knife. He was the owner of a jewelry store. The attacker walked in, and the attacker and the store owner then exchanged words. The bad guy pulled out a knife and the fight began. For the first thirty seconds or so, the store owner seemed to be winning. He was able to get a two-on-one grip on the bad guy's knife-hand. He was able to administer a few knees and kicks. He was going forward, which put the bad guy on his heels and in a defensive posture. All of a sudden, within seconds, the store owner's momentum shifted. He let go of the weapon and he turned his back to try to run for the door. When he turned his back, the bad guy was able to land several stabs to the upper back and rear neck. It was a horrible thing to watch. As I studied the video footage, I asked myself why the store owner would stop doing what he was doing to the bad guy when his strategy was working. I then realized a couple of noticeable things. One, the store owner was overweight, and the bad guy looked to be in fairly good condition. Two, the store owner, after thirty seconds of defending himself, became obviously fatigued. At that point, the fight shifted and he had no choice but to try and flee. In doing so, he gave up his advantage and, unfortunately, was defeated.

At one point, I noticed that a lot of students who were training at my studio were starting to come to class about ten to fifteen minutes late. The reason was that they were skipping the warm-up. The warm-up generally involves conditioning exercises. I've had students tell me that they had no interest in the conditioning portion of classes and that they were only interested in learning Krav Maga. I explained to them that the class is an hour long. How can they learn Krav Maga in a one-hour class if they are only able to last the first fifteen minutes? *"I don't fear the guy that knows 500 kicks, I fear the guy who has done one kick 500 times,"* — Bruce Lee. How can you do one kick 500 times if you get fatigued after the fiftieth kick or even just the fifth?

In boxing, the warm-up may take anywhere from thirty minutes to an hour. There is rope jumping, road work (road work is what boxers call jogging), push-ups, sit-ups, shadowboxing — all that before you have thrown or blocked one punch. Conditioning beats class. I have seen plenty of competitive fights both in the ring, in the cage, and in the streets where one guy who was clearly more skilled was eventually dominated by a less skilled opponent, all because the less skilled opponent was in better shape and the skilled opponent got fatigued. Fatigue makes cowards of us all.

Avoidance is also a huge reason for getting yourself into great shape. Remember, it is better to avoid a violent encounter in any way possible than to have to engage in one. It is a known fact that predators prey on the weak or at least those they think are weak. The weaker you appear, the more likely you are to be preyed upon. I don't know if Vin Diesel is actually a good fighter, but I also don't know of many people who would take the chance of finding out. Sometimes, you just have to look the part.

"In truth, we are not just fighting the bad guys. We are fighting diabetes, cardiovascular disease, cancer, and a long list of other conditions that are the result of a lifestyle that is not focused on health and fitness. To be effective with self-protection and to be able to apply martial arts skills, we need to include real fitness in our training." Tactical Arts Academy.

You have to get in shape. Not only does getting into shape increase your chances of survival in a self-protection situation, but it also increases your chances of having a longer, healthier, more prosperous life.

Then there is the mental factor. If you take care of your body, then your mind will work better as well. Your best weapon will always be the six inches between your ears. Remember, mind, body, and spirit are all connected when it comes to self-protection. Just like the theme song from the hit sitcom Married with Children says, *"Like in love and marriage. They go together like a horse and carriage. This I tell you, brother. You can't have one without the other*

:). "Oh, and by the way, I hear Al Bundy in real life is a Jiu Jitsu Black Belt :).

Commandment #5

Embrace the suck

I remember a story that was told by world champion point fighter Jadi Tention. Jadi is no ordinary fighter. He is not only extremely gifted; he is also very hardworking. Hard work beats talent when talent doesn't work hard. When talent works hard, the result is a champion. Jadi is unquestionably a champion. He lived in the Bronx, and he had just started taking Jiu Jitsu classes. Everyone knew him as a world champion, but he was new to BJJ. During one of their rolling (sparring) sessions, he heard the instructor shout out, "Hey, Jadi! You suck!" At first, he didn't think that he heard the instructor properly, and then a second time, he yelled out, "Jadi, you suck!" Jadi, like myself, has an eccentric and joking personality, so he thought he was just trying to be funny. The instructor repeated it a third time, this time with more focus, "Jadi, I mean it. You suck!" After the session, he felt as though the instructor was purposely putting him on the spot because of his credentials, but that was not the case. "Jadi," his instructor said to him, "You are one of the greatest point fighters of all time, but you suck at Jiu Jitsu. You suck because you're supposed to suck. You're new. The only way to improve at Jiu Jitsu or anything else in life is to be comfortable in embracing the suck."

Be brave enough to suck at something new. Anonymous

A black belt is just a white belt that didn't quit. A black belt is someone who has learned to embrace the suck. Most people cannot embrace the suck. Most people will not become black belts, nor will they be able to become proficient in the art of protection and self-protection. To do so, you have to be willing to accept the fact that you don't know what you are doing. You have to be willing to learn. Most importantly, you have to learn to enjoy the process.

After boxing for my entire adolescent and teenage years, I wanted to focus more on Taekwondo, particularly the sports Karate point fighting. As a boxer, you always fight with your strong side to the rear. I am right-handed, so I lead with my left side forward. In sports Karate point fighting, the goal is to get from point A, where you are, to point B, where your target is, as fast as possible to get the point. Most sports Karate fighters lead with their strong side, which in my case, of course, was my right because it's faster. When I started training with the late great Master

Dawson, the first thing that he said to me was that I needed to change my stance and start leading with my right side forward. This was new to me. I practiced for hours a day, learning how to and being comfortable with fighting as, what we call in boxing, a southpaw. However, that was not the discouraging part. The discouraging part was that I had reached a point in my training where I was not only insufficient at fighting with my right side forward, but I could also no longer fight with my left side forward. I sucked on both sides. Then, I had never felt so vulnerable and incapable of defending myself. When I expressed this feeling to Master Dawson, he told me something that I've never forgotten. "Yes, I know," he said. "This is where most people quit and go back to doing what they are more comfortable with."

This is what Jadi's Jiu Jitsu instructor called "The Suck." This is the bottom of the bench press on the max-out day. This is the first day of your new foreign language class. It's your first day at school. This is how you learn self-protection.

You do have options. You can quit and go back home and never learn to defend yourself or your loved ones, or you can continue to move forward and embrace the suck with the confidence of knowing you will get better.

Commandment #6

You must spar

Okay, let's get down to the nitty-gritty. You must spar. I have a lot of potentially good fighters in some of my beginner-level I classes. Notice I said *potentially* good fighters. I don't allow my students to start to spar until they reach level II, which can sometimes take six months or more. During that time, not only am I teaching the fundamentals, but I am also building their confidence and heightening their fighting spirit. That being said, I don't know just how good they will be or won't be until I see them spar. I don't expect them to be good the first time. What I look for is the fight. They say you can take the dog out of the fight, but you can't take the fight out of the dog. So many students avoid live sparring, especially when there are strikes involved. This is one of the things that makes Jiu Jitsu training so popular. They can train at full speed without having to worry about getting punched. However, when it comes to self-protection training, I feel that this is a dangerous mistake. I like the saying, "Without sparring, it's just dancing."

There is no way to exactly emulate a real attack in practice. You can emulate the movements. You can somewhat emulate the stress, at least the physical stress, but to emulate the sheer violence of an attack is highly unlikely without causing injury to your training partner. The next best thing to emulating a real attack in practice is through sparring.

Sparring is a form of training common to many combat sports. Although the precise form varies, it is essentially relatively free-form fighting with enough rules, customs, or agreements to minimize injuries. This essentially means that you can practice the things that you have learned in your training without trying to hurt or injure someone. As I have repeated a few times in this book, fighting combat is timing and distance. How do you know how close you need to be to land a punch if you've never landed a punch? How do you determine the proper timing and speed to block a kick if you have never blocked a kick? Most importantly, how do you know what a strike feels like if you've never been struck, even lightly?

Often, students spar for the first time fully suited with boxing gloves, headgear, shin guards, and sometimes even body protection, and yet, when they feel the impact of a strike, they freeze. Everything they had practiced for however long they had been training immediately goes out the window. This freeze can cost you dearly in a real situation. If you freeze in a controlled sparring session, you will likely freeze in the streets.

I have sparred with a few of my Jiu Jitsu partners who ordinarily would wipe the floor with me. When we add in strikes, the game changes entirely. Depending on who I am sparring with, the advantage tilts towards my favor. If we add a knife, 95 percent of their techniques are pretty much shut down. Oftentimes, my training partner is sitting there with a confused look on their face. This is the look that you want to have in training, but this is definitely not the look you want to have in a real situation. You need to know what works. You need to know what adjustments to your techniques need to be made. I've seen countless people in different arts spend time on techniques and defenses that would never work in a real or high-speed situation. I would rather they find that out on a mat than in the street.

Now keep in mind that sparring can be dangerous if not done and/or supervised properly. It is very important that you first learn control and establish a set of safety rules between you and your training partner beforehand. If you are training at a good school under a good instructor, these rules will already be established. If you are training on your own, which I don't suggest if you have never sparred before, you need to establish this beforehand. That being said, sparring helps you apply your techniques to real situations. Since a real situation is what we are training for, sparring is a necessity. You must spar.

Commandment #7

Don't fight yourself. Leave that to your opponent.

It's hard enough to go up against your opponent. It's hard enough to identify your attacker's weak points during stress. It's hard enough to train and get in shape to fight. Why add fuel to the fire when there is no need for more fuel?

This happens a lot when you're training and learning new things like how to defend yourself. You start to get frustrated. You start to doubt and even sometimes punish yourself. I often see students do this when they spar with each other. Their opponent will land a punch and instead of shaking it off and moving forward they complain and argue with themselves. They'll say things like, "Oh shit! I should've seen that coming," or "What's wrong with me? I'm better than this." Oftentimes, they even hit themselves as if to say to themselves, "Get it together!" When I see this activity, I always say the same thing. "You're fighting two people, and the one you're losing to is yourself."

You cannot waste time and energy on mistakes that you make during your training or sparring sessions. Once a mistake is made, it is made. There's no need to dwell on it, not even for a second. It only takes a second to make another one, and that's enough time. In a real situation, that could be the fatal one. I often don't like to stop in the middle of my sparring sessions unless we are just drilling some particular techniques. I like to go through the whole round or session and then critique what I did well or could have done. It is similar to typing a document. It is sometimes best to type the whole document and then go back and make your corrections instead of constantly stopping and making corrections as you go. Not only is it frustrating to frequently interrupt your thought process, but it takes longer to finish the document.

This is true for most sports. Although some players, like John McEnroe (a great tennis player), were able to use this to their advantage, they are anomalies. Most players who conduct this type of behavior usually fall short of winning. They even have a name for it: unsportsmanlike conduct. Unsportsmanlike conduct does not only have to be directed at your opponent. Unsportsmanlike conduct can also be pointed back at yourself. A good sportsman won't allow himself to get angry. A good sportsman won't throw his mouthpiece into the stadium. A good sportsman won't damage their hand by hitting the wall or floor when they make a mistake.

To learn something new, including the art of self-protection, we have to understand that although we strive for perfection, we are not perfect. We will make mistakes. You learn from them and you move forward. Contrary to popular opinion, you can make the same mistake twice. In that case, you should learn again and move forward again. Eventually, you will find yourself making the same mistakes less and less.

In Krav Maga, we instill in our students very early on that when we're under attack, the only direction that we go is forward. We do not remain still and we do not move back. Staying still is something you cannot do when you're under attack. If you have to fight multiple opponents, make sure one of them is not you. You have to train yourself to not fight against yourself.

Commandment #8

You must add stress to your training

No matter how long you train, how hard you train, or how many techniques you master, all of your skills will diminish under stress. Let's take swimming, for example. I consider myself an average swimmer. One day, I decided to go for a swim at a local rec center. I thought it would be a good idea to add swimming to my conditioning for my black belt test prep. Once I got to the pool, I was surprised to discover that it was an Olympic-sized pool. I did not know what an Olympic-sized pool meant at the time. An Olympic-sized pool is fifteen feet deep all the way across. I had planned on swimming in a three-to-four-foot deep pool. Needless to say, I was nervous... What if something happened? What if I got halfway and couldn't complete the lap? What if I caught a cramp? All of these thoughts made me seriously consider leaving and going to a reasonable-sized pool. Then I thought to myself, wait a minute. If I can swim across a regular-sized pool, why am I afraid of crossing this pool? After all, water is just water. The answer was stress. Stress has several physical symptoms: exhaustion or trouble breathing, chest pain, or a feeling like your heart is racing, etc. I felt them all. Being able to work under stress is not only important in life but is imperative in a save-your-life situation. You must learn to work under stress.

There are several strategies or techniques for working under stress: learning how to breathe, focusing ahead, and controlling your negative thoughts. However, you will not be able to do any of these if you have never been in a stressful situation. After all, how can you identify with a situation that you have never experienced? Training under stress helps with that identification.

There is no way to directly mimic the feeling or fear of a real violent encounter. But what you can do is mimic some of the symptoms. You can mimic heavy breathing or exhaustion with training drills. For example, doing a series of highly intense aerobic intervals, then immediately working on a technique at full speed. You can mimic the muscle tension or shake by doing a drill that you haven't done before that seems overly difficult. For example, bobbing and weaving punches to the face for the first time with MMA gloves. We have a drill that we call the Gauntlet where a person runs through a group of people as they scream and yell and hit them with pads. The person has to get through the gauntlet and then perform a technique that requires fine motor skills while another group continues to distract them with more yells and strikes. Of course, this drill is done safely and monitored by an instructor, but even in a safe environment, your level of stress increases immensely. You must learn to train and work under stress.

Earlier, I mentioned that you must learn to train at full speed. Training for speed and learning to train under stress is totally different. I can run a full sprint and not feel any stress at all. That same activity with wild dogs running behind me changes things entirely. I can practice escaping a choke hold at full speed with very little stress. Doing that same drill when your training partner is told to not let you out of the choke even if you tap, changes the drill entirely. Light sparring at full speed can only be done by experienced practitioners and has very little stress on an advanced practitioner. Hard sparring with a stranger is entirely different. You must learn to work under stress.

There are a lot of arts that do not include stress in their training. This, in my opinion, does not properly prepare you for competition or a real situation. You need to get comfortable being uncomfortable. Training through stress is also extremely rewarding maybe not during the drill, but when the drill ends, there's no better feeling. It's like facing your fear of swimming across a deep Olympic-sized pool for the first time. Although it is scary, at least you can say you did it and could do it again if you had to.

Commandment #9

Prepare your mind as well as your body.

This is undoubtedly the most important principle/commandment of them all: mindset training. You can be fast and strong with great technique, but without the correct mindset to deal with an actual situation, you will not be well equipped if it were to ever happen. I often tell my students that they're in class for an hour. So, for that hour, it is important that they take their training seriously, stay focused, and train as if the situation is really happening.

What do I mean when I say mindset training? Mindset training is a lot like visualization. Generally speaking, visualization is the process of creating a mental image or intention of what you want to happen or feel in reality. I often train alone because of my schedule. When I am working on a technique or shadowboxing, I visualize a punch, a kick, or a particular attack coming at me, and I respond accordingly. Over the years, I've gotten quite good at it. The mind is a lot more powerful than you may realize. Remember, your strongest weapon is the six inches between your ears. Scientific studies have concluded that visualization can be close to as effective as actual physical training. Such repeated imagery can build both experience and confidence in a person's ability to perform certain skills under pressure or in a variety of possible situations. Mindset training can be just as powerful.

One of the strategies that I used as a sports Karate fighter was visualization. The evening before the event, I would sit back and imagine how the match was going to play out. I imagined my opponents throwing punches and kicks. I imagined the cheering of the crowd. I even imagined what it would feel like when a strike landed. When it was time for the actual match, it was almost like déjà vu. I had been there and done that. My confidence was higher and my abilities were better. My stress levels were also diminished.

When you are training to protect yourself from a real situation, you must put yourself in that situation mentally. The more real you can make the situation in your head, the more prepared your mind will be if the situation were to ever occur. Your mind controls your body. This is the reason why it is sometimes difficult for a person that has been through trauma to go through the actual class. Good self-protection classes deal with real-life scenarios. These scenarios can be triggering for someone that has been through it. Their minds go there automatically and uncontrollably. Working through that trauma is difficult but necessary.

When I tell my students to try to take their class and their training seriously and focus, what I am referring to is for them to imagine that it is not their partner that is standing in front of them but an actual bad guy. To face your fears in the real world, you must first face them in your mind. This does not mean that you can't have lighthearted humor during training. It also doesn't mean that you have to train with a resting stone face the entire session. However, when going through the motions or scenarios, if you can put your mind there, not only will your body follow, but your movements will be more precise.

It is also important that you can release the thoughts in your mind after your training session. Not doing so is the equivalent of going to a horror movie and continuing to think about Freddy when you go home and go to sleep. This is why some people cannot watch horror films. The film is still in their heads even after they are no longer in the theater. When I watch a horror movie at night, I always follow it with a good cartoon before I go to sleep. You must clear the thoughts from your mind after the movie.

This sort of training does not work for everyone that participates in self-protection classes. The reason is that everyone that participates in classes isn't really there to train for self-protection. Some are there to get in good shape. Some are there to interact with their fellow students and friends. Some even find the training to be stress-relieving. *Come here, hit things, feel better* is one of our slogans. All of these reasons are absolutely fine as long as you understand what your reasons are. Some are there for the above reasons and learning to protect themselves just sweetens the deal. And then some are training for self-protection, and the other things sweeten the deal. This brings us to the last commandment.

Commandment #10

Train with a purpose.

As I embark on my Jiu Jitsu training, I have had to embody this last principle: train with a purpose. I have always had a purpose for everything that I have done successfully. I teach because of my love of spreading knowledge. I train because of my desire to be the best I can be. I learned so that I can be a better instructor to my students. Training with a purpose is the same as knowing your why. *Know your why and you'll find your way.* – John C. Maxwell.

Here, however, I would like to dig deeper into what I call "purpose training." Every time you enter your training room, you should have a goal in mind for that particular session. Although your ultimate goal may be becoming a black belt in Jiu Jitsu or Taekwondo, your immediate goal is what you're trying to accomplish on that particular day to get you there. "Today, I'm working on blocking straight punches when I spar." If that's your goal for that particular session, if you get hit by an uppercut or a hook, so what? At least for that session, it's important to defend yourself against straight punches. "Today I am working on retaining my guard position." If someone takes you down, so what? What's important for that particular training session is that you retain your guard as long as possible. Sometimes, my purpose for that day is just to get my ass off the couch and show up for a class on time. No matter what happens after that, at least you made it to class on time.

When you don't have a purpose for your training, you are doing the equivalent of driving without any direction as to where you are going. Yes, you may know where you want to end up, but without having the directions to get there, reaching your destination will be highly improbable. Imagine going to a gym not knowing what body part you're going to exercise on that particular day. What would happen is that you would aimlessly go from machine to machine, never really improving your body. Imagine going to a shopping mall without an idea of what you are looking to buy. You would probably end up with a lot of items that you don't need. I realize that purpose training may not be the most appealing on the surface. There are so many different types of weights in the weight room that you want to try them all. There are so many stores in the mall, and you want to visit them all. There are so many moves and submissions in Jiu Jitsu and you want to perfect them all. However, Rome was not built in a day, but when it was finally built, it became one of the most powerful nations in human history. Perfection takes time.

If you have a good instructor with a well-thought-out curriculum, you won't need to put much thought into your purpose training. Your instructor will do that for you. Every time you come in, they will have a lesson plan for you to follow. That is the benefit of training with a group or even having your own personal coach/instructor. Instead of you trying to create your map, the map has been pre-created for you.

Purpose training also helps you to monitor your progress. If you tilt back and forth from technique to technique, move to move, it will be more difficult to know whether or not you are getting better. When you take one step at a time, it becomes easier for you to look back and see how far you've come. Purpose training is a long game. This is why I lean more toward programs that have curriculum. A curriculum, in my opinion, is a plan of attack. It also helps tremendously when everyone in your training group has the same training purpose. If you're working on hook punches and everyone in the group is working on hook punches, then everyone can help each other grow. However, that is not always the case. It is important that you know your purpose. Sometimes, you can express this purpose with your training partner or partners. Perhaps your purpose will complement theirs. Perhaps you are working on your takedown defenses, not letting anyone knock you off your feet, and your partner is working on takedowns, knocking someone off their feet. This makes for a great training session.

When I was younger, probably around the age of twelve, my dad started teaching me to box. He would take me out to the alley and start to work with me on my punches. I will never forget the first punch I ever learned. It was a left jab. The jab is the first punch that boxers learn. It is done by your lead hand, which is normally your left. It comes out straight and powerful, like the piston of a tractor. The purpose of the jab is to keep your opponent at bay, distract them, and also set up other punches. No good puncher can go without the jab.

Every time we would train, my dad would have me throw jabs up and down the alley, which was about fifty yards long. When I finished, he would say, "Do it again." This went on for every session for at least six months. Finally, I asked him when I was going to be able to learn to throw another punch. His response was, "After you learn this one." His training motto was simple: don't move on to another thing until you have perfected the first thing, purpose train. Those days in the alley weren't very mentally exciting. But to this day, I haven't run into too many people who can stop my jab.

"I hated every minute of my training, but I said, 'suffer now and spend the rest of life as a champion.'" – Muhammad Ali, the Greatest of All Time!

When you purpose train, it's also easier for you to count your wins. Everybody wants to be a winner. If you have no purpose, you will feel as if you're never winning. The reason for this is that you haven't clearly defined what a win means for that day or session. The most successful and fulfilled people in the weight room are always the ones that not only record their workouts but also have a clearly defined goal for that particular day. Last week, they benched 225. Today, their goal is to add on another ten pounds. Once they accomplish that goal, they will increase the weight in the next session. Rinse, recycle, and repeat as they continue to monitor their wins. The most accurate shooters at the gun range are always the ones with a target goal in mind. Last week, they hit their target dead center, at twenty-five feet. This week, they'll move it back a few yards. They may even time their reloads to beat their previous times. They have a goal, and reaching that goal is a win.

It's also important that you set realistic goals. It is not realistic to go from a 225 bench press to a 325 bench press in a week. Nor is it realistic to go from being able to fight off a choke hold from one attacker to be able to handle multiple attackers by your next class. Remember, your purpose is to get one win at a time. Your goals are measurements that help you get there. Set small goals. Small goals add up to big wins. If you're not reaching your small goals, then set smaller ones. Remember that it's your race and you're the only runner. There's no need to rush.

When all is said and done, following these commandments, or even creating your own, will make your journey of learning to protect yourself not only more proficient but more sustainable as well. Sustainability is important. The longer you stick to your training, the better you will become.

Chapter Eleven

Self-Defense (A Legal Term)

I own a school named Krav Maga CDK *Self-Defense Center*. When people ask me what I do, I tell them that I am a self-defense *instructor*. People come to me and tell me that they want to learn *self-defense*. Yet, throughout this book, I have veered away from using the term, "self-defense" and instead, I have used the term, "self-protection." The reason? Self-defense is a legal term.

When it comes to self-protection, there are five important elements everyone should know.

1) Mental preparation: understanding and being willing and capable of using violence to defend yourself.

2). Physical preparation: knowing how to and being capable of physically defending yourself.

3). The actual act: doing what you are trained to do if or when the shit goes down.

4) The psychological aftermath: actually being at peace with what you did. Inflicting violence can give good people nightmares for life.

5). The legal issues: understanding the legal ramifications and consequences of your actions.

I have been training in martial arts for over thirty years and I have never met an instructor that was an expert in all five categories, although I've met some that claim to be.

About ten years ago, I started to think that it was important to learn about the legalities of what I was teaching my students to do. At the time, I was teaching in Washington, D.C., which I soon found out had an entirely different set of laws than that of the state of Maryland, which was pretty much across the street. Maryland has a totally different set of rules from Virginia, which is also in the same vicinity. If that didn't make things complicated enough, the legal jargon that is used in law is pretty much equivalent to reading a foreign language. It is almost written as if you're not supposed to understand. I guess that's why good lawyers get paid so well.

I am an expert when it comes to teaching someone the physical components of protecting themselves against violence. I am not a psychiatrist, nor am I a criminal defense attorney. If you have made the decision that you will defend yourself and your family by any means necessary, there are a few books that I would definitely recommend, including The Law of Self-Defense by Andrew Branca, Force Decisions by Roy Miller, In The Name of Self-Defense by Mac Young, Why Me? by Robert Bryan, and The Gift of Fear by Gavin de Becker. In *this* book, I'll cover some basics.

What is self-defense, really? Self-defense is a legal term used to explain why an individual or group of individuals engage in violence to legally protect themselves, their loved ones, or their property. What that means is that you are supposed to be allowed to use a reasonable amount of force that you deem necessary to defend yourself, defend another person, defend your property, prevent a crime, etc. Let's break this down.

What exactly is a reasonable amount of force? More importantly, who determines it? Well, that's where the jury comes in. If a violent situation is prosecuted under the law, a jury or a judge has to decide whether or not, given the particular circumstances, what the perpetrator did was reasonable. Here's an example: You're standing on one side of a street. Another person is on the other side of the street. That person makes a verbal threat against you, and you respond by pulling out a gun and shooting that person. Yes, the person threatened you, but you would have a hard time convincing the judge or jury that the amount of force you used was reasonable. However, if that same individual was six feet away from you and holding a knife, that same act might be considered reasonable.

When teaching self-protection, most instructors assume their students are good people. They assume that if their students were ever in a situation where they had to use violence to protect themselves, the student would be the good guy, not the bad guy. While this may be true, it is important to remember that self-defense is a *legal term*. Unfortunately, the law doesn't care who the good guy or the bad guy is in a situation. The law cares only about the law.

If a woman is jogging on a trail and a man jumps out of the bushes, attacks her, and attempts to sexually assault her, I don't think there would be too many things that she could physically do that would be considered unreasonable to protect herself. However, there are some things that she could say that, when given to the right prosecutor with the right political agenda, could be used to put her behind bars. Here's an example:

A woman gets attacked while jogging. She can get away, and as she is running, the bad guy starts to chase her. The woman picks up a rock and hits the bad guy in the head; the bad guy falls to the ground and dies. When the police arrive, they ask her what happened. Her response is, "This asshole grabbed me and pulled me into the woods. He thought he would be able to scare me and I would give in. I pushed him away and as I was leaving, he followed me, so I picked up a rock and I crushed it upside the fucker's skull." I know there are a lot of women who would agree with what the jogger did. They would give her the female badge label of a badass.

Believe it or not, good people have gone to jail for a lot less.

But if we change the woman's response, it could change the outcome of the situation. For example, if she tells the police, "This man grabbed me when I was running and pulled me into the woods and tried to rape me. I was able to fight him off and run away. He chased me. Fearing for my life, I picked up a rock and swung it."

What you say CAN AND WILL be used against you in a court of law, which is why *self-defense* is a legal term.

Believe me when I tell you that the law can be complicated and, oftentimes, expensive. There is a common belief that if you were to take someone's life, even if you were the good guy and you acted in self-protection, it would cost you a million dollars to stay out of jail. I'm not sure if that figure is true, but it would cost you something. Not knowing the law is no excuse for breaking the law and definitely will not hold up in a court of law. You must know what you can and cannot do when it comes to protecting yourself. I think it is also important that you are not stuck with analysis paralysis and do not act accordingly if or when the situation arises. That is where your training will come in. Not only your physical training and your mental preparation but also your training as it pertains to the law. It may also help to have a lawyer on retainer. I have self-defense insurance, which although it doesn't cover everything, at least helps me sleep well at night knowing that I have some sort of protection so that I can protect myself or someone else without hesitation.

Most self-protection instructors don't consider the legal aspects of what they are teaching their students to do. Most don't know anything about it. The question is, should they? If they are any good at what they do, then they are teaching their students to think before they react and not react before they think. They should also at least advise their students to know that not only the things they do but also the things they say can incriminate them. Beyond that, they are probably stepping outside their area of expertise, unless, of course, they're a lawyer. It is dangerous to give out legal advice when you're not a lawyer. An instructor is looked upon by his students as an expert in whatever they are teaching. If they are teaching how to punch, their students will view them as experts in punching. If they are teaching how to do a rear-choke, their students will view them as an expert in the rear-choke. If they teach kicks or gun disarms, it's the same deal. If you are not an expert, you shouldn't be teaching that particular subject matter. When I am speaking on a topic or even a technique that I'm not fully trained or qualified to teach, I always preface it with "I'm not an expert on this." I do this often, especially when I'm teaching officers. I teach them gun disarms, for example. Once they take away the gun, they are now out of the area of my expertise. I can shoot, but not nearly good enough to teach how, when, or even why to an officer of the law.

Lawyers go to school for years to be able to understand and make a living doing what they do. There are just as many branches of law as there are martial arts systems. There's tax law, business law, bankruptcy law, constitutional law, family law, estate law, and the list goes on. Just like with martial arts systems, most lawyers don't know squat about the other branches. The last thing you want is to be represented in a murder trial by a medical malpractice lawyer. The last thing you want is to be taught what to say to a police officer in a self-defense shooting by a martial arts instructor. Any self-respecting medical malpractice lawyer would refer you to a good criminal defense lawyer. Any good self-protection/martial arts instructor would do the same. For all my students that are reading this book, if I haven't told you that before, I just did.

Chapter Twelve

Do Black Belts Count in the Streets?

Belt promotions. Do they even matter? Nearly every martial arts system has a belt ranking system to go along with it. Different systems have different belt rankings. The standard is to start with a white belt and end with the infamous black belt. Belt ranking is said to go back as far as the eighteenth century. It is said to have been invented by a great Judo practitioner to properly pair competitors up with one another according to their rank. Then there's the oh-so-famous legend of the Japanese martial artist who would wear a white belt and never clean it. As the belt became old and stained, it would get dark, thus becoming a black belt. Although this is a myth and probably not true, there are many people to this day that never wash their belts.

I remember I used to go to tournaments back in the day and I was always impressed by the Masters who wore dingy old and ragged torn black belts. I thought to myself, "Wow, they must have been training for a long time." When a friend of mine got his black belt, he hung it outside of his car door when he was driving so it would drag down the street and get shredded. When he wore it, people thought he was a master. There are lots of people that dream and fantasize about one day becoming a black belt. My instructor used to say that a black belt was a white belt that had mastered his basics.

What's that all got to do with self-protection? Do you need a black belt to know or be able to protect yourself? Is every black belt really a black belt?

"Karate here." He points to his head. "Karate here." He points to his heart. "Karate never here." He points to his waist. Mr. Miyagi. Karate Kid

I agree with Mr. Miyagi. People are way too concerned about belt ranking. I understand that achieving a higher belt is a great accomplishment. Every time I received a new belt color, I felt honored. A new belt can also symbolize, in physical form, how hard you have worked. Although a lot of people like to deny it, the truth of the matter is that we all like to be recognized. That being said, the color of the belt around your waist will not help you if you find yourself in the unfortunate event of having to physically protect yourself. I have had plenty of beginner-level white belts in my classes that I would much rather be with if I had to protect myself than some of the higher-ranking students. Some students will memorize every technique and will not be able to physically articulate what it would be like in a real situation. I'll take a white belt with the heart of a lion over a black belt with the bite of a puppy any day of the week.

"It's not the black belt that you wear on your waist. It's the black belt in your heart and knowing that you can go out there and you can do it. That's what a true black belt is." – Bonnie Canino

So why are they needed? Although it makes sense when it comes to training for competitions, why even bother to have belts as it pertains to self-protection? Believe it or not, there are some very good reasons for this. One of the reasons that I talk about a lot is the curriculum. Every art has a curriculum. Boxing has the jab, the uppercut, the hook, the footwork, the bobbing and weaving, etc. Jiu Jitsu has the full mount, open guard, close guard, arm bar, rear naked choke, the triangle, etc. Krav Maga has 360 defenses, inside defenses, handgun takeaways, stick attack defenses, etc. The list goes on, but there's always a curriculum.

If you have a small school or a training location of five to ten students in which you all started together and you are training together, then there's probably no need for a belt system. Years ago, I used to train and teach the kids in my neighborhood. I knew what everyone had learned and what everyone's capabilities and talents were. Even then, it became difficult when a new kid came in to train. I would have to pull him aside and teach him the beginning fundamentals while everyone else worked on skills that we had been going over for weeks or even months. That was only with a handful of people inside of a two-car garage. Imagine a school with 30, 300, or even 3,000 students. When new students come into a school, it is important that they first start with the fundamentals. Although I'm a firm believer in always practicing your basics, at some point in time, a student will need to add more to this skill set. This is the only way that they will be able to challenge themselves and grow, get better, or even just stay interested. This is where the belt system comes in.

Belts help both you and your instructor know where you are on your journey. Imagine starting grade school and on the first day of school, instead of learning addition and subtraction, you start with trigonometry. Why? Because everyone else in the class has already done their adding and subtracting, division, multiplication, and geometry. How long do you think you would last in that class? What about the students that have advanced to trigonometry and go to a class where they have to learn to add and subtract? How interested will they be in that class? Belt levels are necessary.

Some students have told me that they don't care about a belt system, and some have refused to even be part of one. I try to explain to them or ask them, "How do I know what to teach you if I don't know what you already know?" Although I do have several private clients for whom the belt ranking is unnecessary, (unless, of course, they decide to go to another school with a different instructor). That is because they are just training with me. The belt system is designed for a multitude of students. Which is, by the way, why Mr. Miyagi didn't need one. He only had Danielson :).

Unfortunately, just like with everything that becomes popular, money becomes involved and everything goes to shit. Bullshit, to be frank. Here's how it starts: A student walks into a school with aspirations of becoming a black belt. The school owner signs them up and starts them on their journey. The longer the journey, the more money for the school owner. Just like with anything, the student wants to not only feel but also see their progress toward their goal. So, every time the student starts to become uninterested in school, the owner gives him another belt. Then it gets even shadier because pretty soon the school owner will start to run out of belts to promote them with. There was a time when there were only two belts in the original Judo system. Most Jiu Jitsu systems only have five or six. Krav Maga is the same way. However, I have seen schools that have more than thirty belt rankings before you achieve so-called black belt excellence. Why? Because they gotta keep that golden goose laying eggs.

So how do you know if you're being fed shit if you don't know what shit tastes like? Well, I'll give you three red flags to look for.

Number one: Attendance.

If your belt promotion is <u>primarily</u> dependent upon how many classes you attend, chances are you're being fed shit. Everyone learns at a different pace. You will have those who can learn in just ten classes, while it may take others thirty to understand the same curriculum. When your attendance is the deciding factor on your promotion, you know that it has little to do with your skill set.

Number two: The price tag.

I have been to schools where, when your belt level increases, so does the price of your classes. After all, the higher your belt, the more they are going to teach you, which means the more you should be paying, right? I can tell you firsthand, as an instructor, that this is not true. The hardest students to teach are the beginner students, the white belts. As students begin to grow and learn and understand the basics and body mechanics of what they're doing, they become much easier to teach and they also learn at a faster rate. To be honest, as their belt level goes up, the price should go down. Oh shit! I probably shouldn't have said that. Hopefully, I will remember to delete that sentence :).

Number three: The quality of higher-ranked students.

The higher-ranked students at your school are a direct reflection of what you will become. Are the higher-ranked students proficient or are they not much better than you? When you walked into your school, you had an idea of what you wanted to become. Are your higher-ranked students a reflection of that image? I also think paying attention to the character of your higher-ranked students matters. How do they carry themselves? Are they honorable or are they arrogant? Are they confident or do they come off as deeply insecure? Are they helpful or are they selfish? How does this pertain to self-protection? Like I said before, the way a person carries themselves is directly related to whether they will ever have to defend themselves.

If the answers to all three of these clues come out positive, then the next step is to trust your instructor. This, once again, is why the character of your instructor matters. You should know that your instructor is not going to put you in a situation that you are not prepared for. Since we are training for self-protection, the instructor is not going to make you believe that you can protect yourself in a given situation if you cannot. This is why the person that is teaching self-protection is so important. They are responsible for teaching someone and showing someone how to potentially save their life and the life of another if necessary. This should not be taken lightly.

There are some systems in school that require you to take a test to be promoted to a higher level. Others have belt ceremonies. Then there are those where the instructor, at his or her discretion, will decide that you are ready and will present you with your next belt.

My first black belt.

I will never forget when I received my first black belt. I was a sports Karate fighter with aspirations of becoming a professional. I worked hard to climb up the ranks. Even as a white belt, I would raise money to fund my tournament and travel expenses. In time, I became one step away from the professional rankings of a paid black belt. I was a brown belt. My instructor, Master Dawson, took me to a tournament where I was to compete. When I got to the tournament, he went to the booth to sign me up. I got changed, put on my brown belt, and went to the brown belt ring. The way Karate tournaments work is a competitor in that division fights to elimination until there's only one left. The one competitor left is the champion of that division. Several brown belts were waiting to be called to their prospective ring. During the first-round callouts, I didn't hear my name. No problem, I thought. I must have been given what is called a *by*. A by is when you're automatically sent to the next round because there is no one for you to fight. During the second-round callout, I didn't hear my name. This is when I started to get worried. I said to my instructor, "Something must not be right. They didn't call my name." He assured me that everything would be fine and to just be patient. Third-round callout, no name. Fourth and last round callout, still no name.

At this point, I was sure that a mistake had been made. Was I just supposed to fight the last man standing? Just as I had started to lose faith, Master Dawson walked up to me and said, "Take off the belt." "I knew it," I said to myself. "There was a mix-up and my name wasn't on the list." I took off my belt and seconds later, Master Dawson wrapped my first shiny black belt around my waist. "Here man, go make me proud. You're fighting in the black belt division today." I was honored, in shock, and also extremely worried. Was I ready? Was I going to embarrass myself and my instructor? More importantly, would I get hurt?

These were all the questions that went through my mind but only for a few minutes. Not only did I have the utmost trust in my instructor, I also knew it was time for me to fight. My name was the first name called. I ended up having to fight the top-ranked black belt in the division. In the streets, this would've been the perfect example of a type two unplanned fight. That being said, when it's go time, it's go time. Get right or get left! As it turned out, I did well. Although I did not win, it was a very close match that even went to what we call sudden death, where the next point wins. I was ready. I did not embarrass myself, my school, or my instructor. I didn't get hurt. My instructor was right. (Later on, I still had to take the actual black belt exam, but my first belt still meant the most.)

Becoming a true black belt can be a great accomplishment. It means you're a badass. A badass is someone who never quits, who fights through adversity, who sets a goal and sticks to it until the end. Only one out of every 200 students that enter a martial arts studio will become a black belt.

Being a black belt is a state of mind and attitude. Even though surrounded by several enemies set to attack, fight with the thought that they are but one.

Morihei Ueshiba

That is what works in the streets.

Chapter Thirteen

Can My Child Learn Self-Protection?

When parents call me and request to enroll their child in my school, I always ask them the purpose or motivation for getting their child into the program. The most common response is that they want their child to be able to defend themselves. My next question is, "Defend themselves against who?" Do they want their child to be able to defend themselves against Butch the Bully in their third-grade class, or are they thinking about their eleven-year-olds being able to defend themselves during a potential kidnapping? This is where reality and honesty must step in. The reality of the situation is that no matter how many years or how skilled an eighty-pound eleven-year-old may be, the chances of fighting off a 200-pound grown man are a hundred to one.

Now, of course, there's always the lucky surprise kick to the groin and the running for your life technique, which we all teach, but far from that, there's not much more that they can do once contact has been made.

Once contact is made, it is what we call the "Right side of Bang." _Left of Bang,_ on the other hand, is another story, and a pretty good book by the way. Being left of bang means avoiding or getting away from a situation before contact is made. If you are concerned about your child being the victim of an asocial violent situation by an adult, which you should be, then physical self-protection is not where you should put your money. (An asocial violent attack refers to being attacked by a stranger). Your child needs to learn about:

Focus and what to focus on.

Awareness and what to be aware of.

Stranger danger.

Where is the exit and which way is home?

How to use their voice.

Run, hide, yell, etc.

If this is your primary concern, look for an instructor that can answer these questions and knows how to instill those answers into your child.

Then there's Butch the bully. No matter the age of your child, if they are old enough to attend school, then they have met Butch the bully. They may not have told you, but he's there and everyone at the school or in the neighborhood knows who he or she is. There's a Butch the Bully in preschool. There's a Butch the Bully in kindergarten, middle school, junior high school, high school, and college. There are even Butch the Bullies in the adult workplace. Butch the Bully can live at the same address as you. This brings us back to our regularly scheduled program and the question, "Can my child learn self-protection?"

I made a video on YouTube called *Krav Maga versus Taekwondo*. This video broke down which martial arts system I think is best for which age group. In my opinion, for ages twelve and below, the more traditional martial arts systems, including Taekwondo, Karate, Kung Fu, etc., are best. For ages twelve to sixteen, the more assertive systems are best: Krav Maga, Jiu Jitsu, boxing, and even wrestling. Once they reach the age of sixteen, they can then make their own decision. Let me explain the reasons for my thoughts.

The definition of martial is 'of or appropriate to war, war-like.' The definition of art is an experience consciously created through an expression of skill or imagination, a method of way. This means martial art, by definition, is the way an individual or group of people express themselves during war, or in this case, a fight. So, the real question you have to ask is how you would want your child or teen to express themselves in a fight that they could not avoid. Now, of course, this will always depend on the situation, but generally speaking, what would be your answer?

You have to be very careful when you're putting your child into a school of combat. This is why I recommend that kids start in the more traditional programs. Your traditional programs focus more on the behavioral aspects of martial arts: courtesy, integrity, perseverance, indomitable spirit, self-control, etc. When a child is instilled with these tenets, confidence comes along with the package. Confidence is the biggest and best weapon against Butch the Bully. Confidence to Butch is like kryptonite to Superman. As they get older, Butch gets bigger, badder, and more resilient to kryptonite. This means that for your child to protect themselves against Butch, they need to be more resilient and assertive.

Still, a great amount of restraint should be warranted. A teenager isn't expected to understand control. I even have adults that don't know their strengths. A teenager isn't expected to be able to make the best decisions and fully understand the consequences of their actions. This is why in our justice system, you're not tried as an adult in most court cases until you are eighteen years of age, and once you become eighteen, mistakes that you made previously normally get expunged.

You want to teach your child that there is a time to fight and protect themselves and there is a time not to. But when it is time, you want them to know how. When I teach adults, I concentrate on one situation only: an asocial violent encounter. This is a fight when there is no flight available. I teach them to inflict injury over pain, to incapacitate their attacker, and do what is necessary to get home safe. For obvious reasons, this is not what I teach my teens. They are more likely to have to deal with a social violent situation (a social violent situation refers to someone you know). I teach my teens to address the immediate danger. Attack or counterattack as needed and get away as soon as they can, hopefully without injuring or permanently maiming Little Sassy Sarah or even Butch. The last thing any good instructor wants is to get a phone call from his thirteen-year-old student's mother telling them that the child got into a schoolyard debate and now the other kid is in traction from a move they taught him.

Another reason for my opinion is that a lot of traditional martial arts schools are physical but are not as violent. Systems like Jiu Jitsu, wrestling, and Aikido are great examples. These arts focus on controlling Butch and Sarah, but not hurting them.

At the end of the day, it comes back to the instructor. Who is the instructor? Is he Sensei Kreese or Mr. Miyagi? To be quite honest, as we are finding out from the recent seasons of "Cobra Kai," the Netflix series, a little bit of both is required :).

Have your child take a class or two with the instructor. See if there's a good connection. Ask the head instructor what their views are on discipline, restraint, and control. If you decide to enroll your child in a course or school, monitor their behavior. Are they more confident but not cocky? Are they more assertive but not disruptive? Are the lessons positively affecting them? If not, take your child out of the course immediately. There are too many good instructors and schools for kids around for you to settle for a bad one. At the end of the day, kids tend to mimic what they see and who they admire. They will admire their martial arts/self-defense instructor. If their instructor carries themselves with great character, then students will also carry themselves that way.

"There is no such thing as a bad student, only bad instructors." — Mr. Miyagi

Chapter Fourteen

Treat Everybody Like Mike Tyson

I was recently speaking to one of my students about the benefits of being nice and kind to people. His response was true, but worth a discussion. He said, "It is a lot easier to NOT be nice than to be nice when someone does something to piss you off." When you're not in a good or friendly mood or when you're having a bad day, being nice is the equivalent of not being sincere, and that takes practice. Another student I have has terrible road rage. Not only did she have road rage when she was driving, but she also had it just walking down the street. If she saw someone else speeding down the street, she felt as though she had to yell at them and set them straight. This particular student was a female, in her fifties, probably around 5 feet 1 inch. What I explained to both of them was essentially the same.

I drew out a scenario. They yelled at that person that was driving recklessly down the street, or they were being mean to a person because they weren't in a good mood. That person decided they weren't going to just continue to drive by or walk away. They decided to stop the car, get out of the car, and confront them with not just words but with an all-out attack. The person decided to use strikes and punches instead of just walking away or confronting them with words. They would be in a fight that, according to street law, they started.

Pushing the envelope even further, imagine if it was Mike Tyson. Mike Tyson, in his prime and probably even today, was one of the most feared human beings on the planet. To this day, if you saw Mike Tyson walking down the street, a chill would probably go through your spine. The reason is that you know what Mike Tyson is capable of doing and willing to do if you rub him the wrong way. What would you do if that were Mike Tyson? Imagine you were driving down the street and you pulled up behind a car at the red light and the light turned green. The car didn't start moving immediately. You're not having a good day, but the person in the car in front of you happens to be Iron Mike Tyson, former heavyweight champion of the world, and you knew it. Would you honk your horn? Would you say "Hey move your f@#kin ass out of the way?" Or would you suck it up and wait patiently for Mr. Tyson to move forward? What if you're standing on the subway and every five seconds someone walks past and bumps into you without saying a word? You're not having a good day. You just lost your job. You're fed up. You say to yourself, "The next person that bumps into me, I'm going to give them a piece of my mind." Five seconds later, a hard bump happens. You look up and you see Mr. Tyson, facial tattoo and all, looking right through you. Do you give him a piece of your mind or do you simply say, "Oh hey Mike," with a smile on your face? Treat everybody like you would treat Mike Tyson.

There are also benefits to treating everybody like you would treat Mike. Treating everybody like you would treat Mike can stop you from getting yourself into unnecessary situations that you could've avoided or walked away from. In certain neighborhoods and certain environments, treating everyone like they would treat Mike is the norm. The only time you don't is when you're looking for a fight. In the prison system, for example, no matter how big or small another prisoner may be, treating them like you would treat Mike may prevent you from having to either take a life or have your life taken. Learn to respect everyone and more people will respect you.

Stop picking your opponents

One of the things that happens a lot in combat sports such as boxing or MMA is that fighters get criticized for picking their opponents. Picking your opponent is what a fighter would do when he's trying to have a good fighting record, trying to make his way to a championship bout, or even trying to remain the champion the easy way. One of the many famous scenes in the Rocky Balboa series is when Rocky decides to fight the gruesome Clubber Lane. He told Mickey that he wanted to have one more fight. Mickey, Rocky's trainer, told them that he could not win against the gruesome Clubber Lane. The reason why he felt that Rocky could not win was that all of the fights that Rocky had won were setups. He put Rocky up against competitors that he knew Rocky could defeat. When you pick your opponents in the boxing or MMA world, you are considered a coward. The fighters that get the most respect are the ones that are willing to fight everybody. Those fighters became fan favorites. The reason is that courage and confidence are admired by everyone. Those are also the same fighters that end up punch drunk by the end of their careers. In the streets, they end up dead.

When I was younger, one thing that got under my skin was when guys on the streets would pick fights with some dudes and back down from fights with others. If one particular guy yelled at them, they were ready to fight, but if another guy that they thought was more dangerous did the same thing, they would suck it up and just walk away. That's called picking your opponents. Here's my suggestion: Try treating everyone the same. If there is a bigger person or a smaller person, man or woman, black or white, treat everyone the same. If you are going to be mean to one person, be mean to everybody. If you are going to be nice to one person, be nice to everybody. Make a decision. Keeping with the subject of self-protection, that decision should lean more to the nicer side. That's the side that may keep you out of jail or even above ground. That doesn't mean that you have to walk up to everybody smiling and grinning (that's not a smart defensive thing to do either). Just treat people with respect. If you have to wonder how to go about doing that, **treat everybody like you would treat Mike Tyson.**

Chapter Fifteen

Beware! The One You Know

Earlier in this book, I mentioned that I would only speak about things that I have seen, witnessed, or experienced myself. Let me tell you a situation that I have experienced. I had a student that we will call Karen. Karen joined my school right after one of the Christmas breaks. Right away, I saw great potential in her development. One of the things that struck me was not only her intensity but her dedication. Unlike most students that are beginners, she seemed to comprehend what we were doing. She understood violence. After a couple of months of training, my instructors and I noticed something that was of concern. Karen would ask questions that were more explicit and descriptive than the average student would ask. She asked questions about two hand chokes where she was being lifted off of the ground. Was there a safe way to jump out of a moving car? How to take a punch, etc. Her questioning prompted me to pull her aside after one of the evening classes to inquire about her motivation. I was not prepared for her response. Right away, Karen burst out into tears and started to explain and describe to me what was going on in her home. She was being domestically abused. She explained that the abuse had started verbally, then graduated to physical, and now had escalated to what she thought was life-threatening. She told me how her partner would regularly threaten her with weapons; knives, sticks, and even guns. She told me she had escape plans and an exit route in case she had to flee for her life. She had decided to take Krav Maga so that she could defend herself, not against a stranger but against her husband.

This was something that I had only heard things about at that time in my career, but I had never experienced them that closely. I did not know if this had happened to one of my students in the past. It was like a movie. My only advice to her was to leave the relationship as soon as possible. I asked her if she had seen the movie, "Enough". Enough is a movie starring Jennifer Lopez. In the movie, she was going through the same thing, and she took Krav Maga for the same reason. I told her about the movie, hoping to inspire her to get away before something bad or even fatal happened.

A few weeks later, as I was teaching one of my classes, two detectives came into the studio and asked to speak with me. I had no idea what they wanted to speak to me about, but when detectives show up at your workplace, it is usually not a good thing. They asked me if I knew Karen and if I had information about the situation. As soon as I heard Karen's name, I accidentally said out loud, "Oh my God, he killed her." The detective looked at me in surprise and said, "What made you say that?" I told them the story. Afterward, they informed me that Karen's husband was dead and Karen had shot him in the head in what she was claiming was self-defense. I was the only one she had confided in about her situation.

When I was growing up, if you had something that was stolen from you, the general assumption was that it was stolen by someone you knew. Unfortunately, violent encounters are no different. But this is not an assumption. Here are the facts:

According to Statista, most victims know their attacker, and the data backs this up. In 2018, very few murders were committed by strangers. The same goes for rape and sexual assault victims; the majority were perpetrated by acquaintances, intimate partners, or relatives. What do we mean when we say stranger or non-stranger? A stranger is classified as an offender they did not see, recognize or know by sight. In other words, a stranger is someone you have never seen before. A non-stranger is classified as an offender who is either related to, well-known, casually acquainted or someone that you recognize. The creepy dude that stays on the corner that you've seen only once or twice would be categorized as a non-stranger.

Then there's domestic violence and dating violence. They are different as well. Domestic violence is any form of abuse that takes place in any relationship. Dating violence is any form of abuse that takes place in a dating relationship.

In 2020 alone, about 141,778 women in the United States were raped or sexually assaulted by well-known or casual acquaintances. So, what does this mean? Get ready and brace yourself for the answer. <u>Your husband, live-in partner, or boyfriend is statistically more dangerous than the stranger lurking in the woods that you've been preparing for.</u>

No one, no matter what they have done, deserves to be abused, especially by someone they love.

I cannot begin to tell someone how to protect themselves from the one they know. I cannot honestly give you techniques or even strategies that will mentally prepare anyone for such a horrific experience. I can teach you to be aware of your surroundings and what to look for when you're out in public or even in a strange place like a movie theater, a restaurant, or a bar (don't go to bars). However, those same strategies don't work when you're in a safe place in your own home. Yes, taking a martial art or a good self-protection system will definitely help, but as I said before, the most dangerous strike in any system is the one you don't see coming, and that holds for the most dangerous attacks as well, and this is an attack you probably didn't see coming or, worse yet, didn't want to see coming.

One of the most popular thoughts when it comes to this type of situation is, "Why didn't they see it coming?" What about the red flags? Why didn't they just walk away or get out of the situation before it got really bad? I find it hard to believe that after all of these years and countless studies on domestic and dating violence, there are still people that believe that walking away is an easy answer. Yes, it is the best answer, but definitely not the easiest one. Although it may be for some, for the ones that fall victim to the situation, it is a lot more complicated. This brings me to my next story and experience.

I had another student who joined my studio years after Karen. Let's give her the name Rhonda. Rhonda, just like Karen, was an extremely dedicated student. She rarely missed a class. She paid attention, she worked hard, and she asked a lot of questions. Unlike Karen, it didn't take a couple of months to find out what her motives were for wanting to take Krav Maga. Rhonda told me her story the first time we met. Rhonda was in a highly toxic relationship. She was married to a man who was physically, emotionally, and verbally abusive. She feared for her life. To make matters worse, Rhonda had a child from a previous relationship. Although she wasn't sure, she was afraid that her child was being abused as well. By that time, I was more experienced as an instructor. By that time, I knew that if she was attacked by her husband, there would be very little that she could do without the situation ending in a possible fatality. I even reluctantly told her about Karen, who, by the way, was charged with murder and is still in prison today. Her response was one that has inspired me and kept me going, even with all the naysayers claiming bullshit when it comes to martial arts/self-protection training. It made me realize what it is that I do. She said to me, *"I am not here for you to teach me how to defend myself against my husband. I am here to build the strength and confidence that I need to leave."*

When I said earlier that learning self-protection and martial arts would definitely help, I was not referring to physical defense. What I was referring to was the self. There is a less than 15 percent chance that my students will ever have to use any of the physical techniques that I teach them. That percentage drops down to maybe five or lower the longer that they stay and train. The reason for this is that they're building up themselves. Their self-esteem, self-worth, self-preservation, self-confidence, and also their self-respect. Why don't they leave? Because they don't have enough "self." Now, please don't think that I am claiming that martial arts is the silver bullet to cure all domestic violence. Nor am I claiming that it will give everyone the "Self" that they need. What I have seen with my own eyes is that it helps. I have seen countless numbers of females walk into my studio with clear low self-esteem issues and walk out with the posture of a queen. I have seen countless numbers of teenagers, who walk in with their heads down, arms folded, hunched over with a clear lack of confidence, walk out with the fighting spirit of a lion. I've seen men who were emasculated by a society, whose self-respect and self-worth had begun to or had already dwindled, walk out of the studio with the swagger of a king. Any good self-defense/self-protection/martial arts instructor will state the same.

So, what happened to Rhonda?

After about six weeks of training with Rhonda, I started to get concerned. I hadn't seen or heard from her in a couple of weeks. This was unlike Rhonda. She rarely missed a day. She would always show up for class. She would have her daughter with her, sitting on the side doing her school-work. I felt the school had become her safe place. I opened my mail one morning to find an unmarked letter from Rhonda.

Dear DJ,

I would like to thank you and your staff for all that you do. Your training has helped me more than you will ever know. Unfortunately, I will need to cancel my membership. The good news is that I've taken my daughter and I've left my husband. We have moved out of state and we're currently staying at a shelter at an undisclosed location. We have a hard road ahead of us, but training at CDK has given me the confidence and strength that I needed to keep moving forward. I now know that I/we will survive and be okay.

Love and thanks

Rhonda

So, I think the question was **<u>Self-Defense. Why even bother?</u>**

The answer

That's why! And that's why I do what I do.

DJ Stephens

Proud self-defense/self-protection/martial arts instructor

THE END

About The Author

DJ Stephens was raised in Washington, D.C. during the late eighties and nineties, at a time when the city was ranked amongst the most dangerous cities in the country. Having been raised in that situation, he was no stranger to violence. Knowing how to protect himself was a necessity for his survival. His first experience with martial arts was at the first Jhoon Rhee Self-Defense Institute in Washington, D.C. He also trained privately with several local black belts. He soon went on to train as an amateur boxer under his father, who was a well-known boxing coach. He trained for several years in Hapkido and received his first black belt in Taekwondo under Master Gerald Dawson. With a desire to train more adults, he found Krav Maga, an Israeli self-defense system. He trained every day for several hours, and within just a few years, he became an expert-level practitioner and the head instructor at The

Krav Maga Institute in Washington, D.C. He is the first Afro-American to receive his Krav Maga black belt in the state of Maryland. Everything he has ever learned, he has gone back to teach others. He has trained boxers, body-builders, MMA fighters, and more. He is the founder of CDK Self Systems LLC, a training system that teaches, motivates, and empowers its students to be confident and strong, push forward during times of stress, and fight until the end. His motto is to save the world one punch at a time through the teachings of self-defense.

" We don't just train warriors. We create them!"

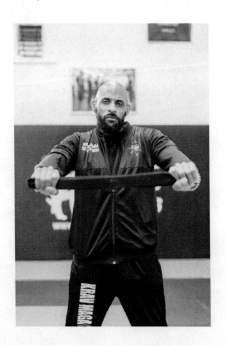

Made in United States
Cleveland, OH
14 March 2025

15149020R00096